MOVE

HOW TO MAKE EXERCISE HAPPEN - YOUR WAY

SARAH ASPINALL

authors
AND CO.

DISCLAIMER - NO MEDICAL OR PERSONAL ADVICE

The information in this book, whether provided in hardcopy or digitally (together 'Material') is for general information purposes and nothing contained in it is, or is intended to be construed as advice. It does not take into account your individual health, medical, physical or emotional situation or needs. It is not a substitute for medical attention, treatment, examination, advice, treatment of existing conditions or diagnosis and is not intended to provide a clinical diagnosis nor take the place of proper medical advice from a fully qualified medical practitioner. You should, before you act or use any of this information, consider the appropriateness of this information having regard to your own personal situation and needs. You are responsible for consulting a suitable medical professional before using any of the information or materials contained in my Material or accessed through my website, before trying any treatment or taking any course of action that may directly or indirectly affect your health or well being.

CONTENTS

"The body is a sacred garment.

It's your first and last garment;

it is what you enter life in and

what you depart life with,

and it should be

treated with honour."

Martha Graham

For Omar, Jemima and Lawrence.
My world.

ABOUT THE AUTHOR

As the founder of Breaking Ballet, Sarah helps busy women prioritise their health and fitness using short and effective ballet-inspired workouts, along with the latest transformational mindset coaching techniques.

As a trained dancer, registered ballet teacher, and certified NLP, Time Line Therapy and Hypnosis practitioner, Sarah's mission is to empower women to develop strong, toned bodies, at the same time as finally allowing themselves the time and space they need to achieve the future they desire with ease and clarity.

With a thriving community of over 18,000 women across 22 countries, Sarah has changed the lives of more than 1000 women through her online membership and group programme. She is a former lawyer, based in the UK, and a mum of two children.

FOREWORD

I love Sarah's approach to movement - and the way she helps people to overcome those barriers that get in the way of moving more or moving differently. Sarah recognises that the greatest barrier to movement is not our body, but our mind.

As a scientist I have spent over 25 years studying the science and psychology of movement and dance. What I found is that humans are born to move and dance and that individuals and societies function better when they move and dance. Movement and dance stimulate four areas of human behaviour: Social, Thinking, Emotional and Physical.

Social: moving together bonds people together. Movement is a social glue.
Thinking: moving changes the way people think. Movement is a cognitive modifier.

Emotional: movement changes the way people feel. Movement is an emotion-communicator.

Physical: movement changes our physical make up. Movement is a whole-brain workout.

Movement is at the heart of effective human behaviour and human functioning. However, there is a problem. I think almost everyone knows that moving more and moving differently is good for our physical and mental wellbeing. Yet despite this knowledge, we live in a sedentary world with high levels of poor physical health and low levels of mental wellbeing. To improve their physical and mental wellbeing people know they need to move more and move differently - and yet they still lead sedentary, unhealthy lives.

Why?

It's all to do with mindset.

Thousands of academic research papers have shown that mindset is the greatest barrier to being physically active - and therefore being physically, emotionally, cognitively and socially healthier. If we want to move more, or move differently, we need to change our mindset.

This is where Sarah's practical book and guide comes in - and it fits perfectly.

Move clearly describes how to change your mindset and overcome the barriers that get in the way of moving more and moving differently. In this brilliant and essential book Sarah lays out a step-by-step guide for how to move your mind – to help you move your body.

So, if you want to move more – start by exercising your mind. *Move* is a fabulous place to start.

Dr Peter Lovatt
Director: Movement in Practice
Author of The Dance Cure

1

THINK BEFORE YOU MOVE

We all know exercise is a vital part of living a healthy life, whether it's for weight loss, heart health, increased energy, strength and tone, mental wellbeing, or simply to feel great.

But many women lack motivation to exercise on a regular basis, or at all. There just seem to be so many barriers preventing us from doing it, or so few opportunities throughout our week to be consistent enough to see results from our efforts.

We are also bombarded with information on social media, in magazines, and from well-meaning friends about the latest fitness fad or which fitness programme is right for us. We are told what it is we really *"should"* be focusing on and how we can achieve our dreams if we sign up now and simply do as they tell us. Different experts or studies tell us different - sometimes conflicting - things about how to be fit and healthy.

It is overwhelming and with the best will in the world, once the confusion sets in, we give up and decide we will start again at some point in the future, when life is calmer and we have more time to figure it all out.

I have been there and I completely understand the challenges you face when you have no time to fit exercise into your hectic schedule, have no energy, no stamina, have lost your body confidence and feel completely overwhelmed.

Then we throw guilt into the mix. We women are fabulous at feeling guilty for prioritising our health and wellness over household chores, childcare, work, or spending time with friends and family.

You may have tried various fitness regimes, but have not stuck to it for any length of time, either because you didn't see the results you were hoping for, or perhaps life simply got in the way and you stopped. And if you're honest, exercise is just not something you enjoy doing!

Cue the negative self-talk – berating yourself for being hopeless, lacking willpower, and allowing your healthy eating habits to go out of the window. You tell yourself you will have to get a grip at some point when the time is right but now things are too busy, too complicated, you are juggling too many things and you can't cope with another task on your to-do list. It's hugely frustrating, but you promise yourself that this time will pass and you will sort it out eventually.

Then you see other women who seem to be working out regularly with ease, so why can't you do it? You ask yourself,

"What's wrong with me? Why can't I sort myself out?" You are momentarily embarrassed, but you dismiss these feelings because that woman you saw doesn't have kids, or doesn't work the hours that you do, so of course she has the time to commit to exercising. It's ok for her because she is not living your life and if she did, she wouldn't have time to workout either.

THERE IS AN EASY WAY TO START

The good news is you are not alone. So many women I speak to have had similar experiences that leave them feeling overwhelmed and unsure what to do next in order to change things - especially, it seems, when we are in our late 30s and beyond. Age is perceived to be an additional barrier to exercising and optimising our health. Countless women have asked me if they are too old to start exercising – if it's just too late to really make a difference to their lives; whether, now they have aches and pains, or arthritis, or injuries that limit their capability to move their bodies as they once did, they should just forget about exercising and focus on other areas of self-care instead. It was after being asked this question by a 35-year-old woman (yes, 35) that I decided to write this book.

WHY IS MOVEMENT SO IMPORTANT?

I know you already appreciate the importance of movement, that's why you want to learn how to make exercise happen for you on a consistent basis, but I think it's worth reiterating some of the basics because this is important when it comes to considering your *"why"* – the reason you want to exercise. After all, that is what motivation is – your *reason* for doing something. It's also important to have an understanding of how important exercise becomes as you enter perimenopause and menopause.

At the time of writing this book, I am 45 years old and well into the throes of perimenopause. In my view, it's one of the most important times in our lives to be moving. Our bodies are experiencing a number of changes that may be uncomfortable and sometimes painful. Exercise can help us through this phase of life and leave us feeling better than ever.

Heart disease

The changes to our bodies as we go through perimenopause and menopause means we are at a higher risk of heart disease. Heart disease is the number one killer of women in the UK. In fact, coronary heart disease kills more than twice as many women as breast cancer. There are currently more than 3.5 million women in the UK living with heart disease and, sadly, 77 women die from a heart attack every day in the UK – around 28,000 women every year[1]. When we hit menopause, this risk increases. A dip in oestrogen levels is common at the onset of menopause. This dip increases the risk of the coronary arteries narrowing, whereas our oestrogen previously protected the lining of the artery walls, reducing the build-up of plaque.

Bone health

Menopause is also an important moment in a woman's bone health. Oestrogen is important for keeping bone density stable and maintaining bone strength. The decrease of oestrogen during perimenopause means bone density starts to go down too.[2] With this loss of bone density comes reduced bone strength and a greater risk of breaking bones. The good news is that working out can help build and maintain bone density.

Muscle mass

In our 40s, we also lose muscle mass twice as fast as men and most of the loss occurs in our core muscles, which support our abdomen. Increasing our muscle mass through bodyweight training helps increase our metabolism and our strength (which in turn supports bone health).

Weight

At this age, we are also more prone to putting on weight around our mid-section and belly fat has been linked to diseases such as diabetes, heart disease, dementia, and certain cancers. Weight loss is also one of the most cited reasons by women for wanting to exercise in the first place, so that they can once again feel confident and comfortable in their clothes.

Mind-body connection

This is where it gets interesting to me as a dancer. Exercise helps to foster a strong mind-body connection. You will have heard the phrase "strong body = strong mind", and in Chapter 12, we will take a deeper look at a revolutionary new understanding of the mind /body connection, revealing how our thoughts and emotions don't just happen inside our heads. The way we move has a profound influence on how our minds operate. This opens up the possibility of using our bodies as tools to change the way we think and feel.[3]

Menopausal symptoms

During menopause, women can also experience many uncomfortable symptoms, and exercise can help to:

- reduce your hot flushes,
- help you to manage your weight,
- lift your mood,
- improve your self-esteem,
- help you to sleep,
- reduce anxiety.

Exercise is a form of self-care. It can improve the way you feel by lowering feelings of anxiety and depression. It can help to manage your stress levels (decreasing your cortisol levels), lift your mood, and clear your mind.

All this means menopause could arguably be one of the most important periods to stay in shape. But this is your personal journey and this book is going to help you discover *your* reason for exercising and how to make it part of your everyday life. Not mine. Not your best friend's, and not other women who are a similar age to you. There is no right or wrong reason and no reason is more *worthy* than the next. As long as the reason is important to you, that is all that matters.

HOW TO MAKE EXERCISE HAPPEN

In the following chapters, I am going to show you how to finally make exercise happen without being overwhelmed, so it becomes part of your lifestyle, not a task on your never-ending to-do list.

I will also show you how exercise can actually be enjoyable while you're doing it, instead of feeling like a punishment for the bag of crisps you ate the night before. Couple this with the benefits to your body of having done the exercise and it's a win-win situation.

I'll teach you plenty of simple strategies to achieve this, but it's not just about the "how". The most important part of your success starts in understanding YOU – your unique personality and what makes you tick. There is no "one size fits all" when it comes to exercise. We need options to choose which kind of approach suits us best. What works for one person doesn't necessarily work for the next. Different things motivate different people. We all respond differently to expectations (both outer and inner expectations) and it's vital that we understand our unique human nature and the reasons behind why we act and why we don't act. I am going to help you work out what these factors are for you, *why* exercise is important to you, and how you can reap the benefits from exercising for just 15 minutes a day.

In this book, you are asked at the end of each chapter to complete tasks to help you gain more self-awareness and to map out your key personal strategies to build and implement goals to create a sustainable habit of exercise. I urge you to complete these tasks as you read through the book. It is the work *you* do that will make the real difference. In the Appendix, I have included a full worked example of what your map to success might look like. You can use this example to help build your own map as you work through the book, or as a reference later on.

We need to remember that there will never be a "perfect" time to make ourselves go through a period of change and therefore, we will have to face inevitable initial discomfort.

I have spent over seven years helping busy women in their late 30s and beyond prioritise their health and wellbeing, using short and effective ballet-inspired workouts and mindset techniques. I am a trained dancer and registered ballet teacher, a mindset coach, and a certified Neuro-Linguistic Programming (NLP), Time Line Therapy, and Hypnosis practitioner.

But it's my many years' experience as a successful lawyer in London, followed by becoming a mum to two children whilst running my fitness business, that have been key in developing my understanding of what really works for us busy women when it comes to creating new habits and prioritising our health and wellness.

I spent 10 years chained to my desk as a lawyer, struggling to find the time to exercise (or frankly, do anything else other than work and climb that corporate ladder). I eventually left my legal career to go back to college to train as a ballet teacher and to raise my two young children while I taught multiple in-person exercise classes a week. At the same time, I was setting up my online business. I have co-taught movement classes to people with Parkinson's Disease and worked with elite board divers in preparation for national competitions, all while navigating motherhood and trying (and more often than I would care to admit, failing) to stay on top of school and home admin. I am busy, just like you. But I LOVE movement and especially dance. I've seen how it can almost magically transform people suffering with Parkinson's Disease from being unable to control their movements to flowing gracefully and with joy. Scientists have studied and been amazed by the power of dance to help people who suffer from all sorts of debilitating conditions.[4] I love teaching it, doing it and of course, inspiring others to do the same.

BUT there are still days when I would rather stay in bed, catch up on all the tasks I know I need to do, or meet a friend for breakfast or lunch. However, I know if I don't move, I don't feel good. And I really want to feel good. Not just for me, but for everyone around me. If I haven't moved my body, I'm not good company. If I have moved (even when I don't feel like it), I feel energised, happy, and more balanced.

And this is exactly how you will feel once you unlock the key to consistent exercise. It will not only help you to drop those stubborn pounds, tone and strengthen your body, but it will also leave you feeling energised, comfortable in your clothes, confident, and back in control. Friends will start to comment on your change in mood and even your appearance, leaving you feeling proud and accomplished. You will feel sexy, have found inner peace and a sense of completeness. And best of all, achieving your health and fitness goals allows you to achieve amazing things in other areas of your life. Things that perhaps you didn't have the confidence to even consider before. Anything becomes possible. And this new-found confidence and contentment has a ripple effect on all those around you. You have more energy and patience for your children, your sex life improves, and you become an inspiration for those around you to follow in your footsteps.

I have clients who have experienced all of this.

Erin struggled with her weight her whole life, but was too embarrassed to attend fitness classes because she was very heavy. She has five children and had gained weight with each pregnancy. She found herself too busy to take care of herself. But when she entered her 40s, she didn't like the way she was feeling. Her back was hurting and she had really bad sciatica down her leg. She realised that if she didn't start taking care of herself, she wouldn't have the energy to take care of her family. Since applying my methods, Erin has been exercising regularly for 10-15 minutes daily, her core is stronger, she has dropped the pounds, her pain has disappeared and her friends have asked her what she is doing to get such amazing arms! Erin has realised it's all about living your best life and being physically able to do the things you want to do for the long term.

Karin was advised by her doctor to change her lifestyle. Once she learnt how to incorporate short, daily workouts into her regime, her health improved drastically. Her angina is now on hold and her sciatica and back pain has eased completely. Her flexibility has improved and she feels so much happier as a result. Her wellbeing has soared and she is managing the menopause much better.

When you implement the simple strategies I share with you in the coming chapters, you are helping to future-proof your body, just like Erin and Karin.

GETTING TO KNOW YOU

We will start by exploring what makes you unique. You will get to know yourself and what motivates you on a much deeper level. We will explore how you respond to inner and outer expectations by looking at your personality profile inside Gretchen Rubin's "The Four Tendencies" framework. Your tendency shapes every aspect of your behaviour, so using this framework allows you to make better decisions and become happier, healthier and more productive. This is the basis of the transformation you will achieve.

You will learn why a reluctance and lack of desire to exercise is completely normal. Voluntary physical movement isn't natural and we will look at how to overcome these feelings of resistance by focusing on the enjoyment and necessity of exercise. We will delve into your beliefs to discover if you are being held back from achieving your goals by the stories you are telling yourself about your own health and fitness, your goals, and your likelihood of success. We will transform any limiting beliefs into new beliefs that will assist you in achieving your goals.

We will also look at your values to discover what is important to you about your health and fitness goals. When you have a better understanding of your values, it provides reinforcement to support you in using your capabilities. Most importantly, our values help us to make sense of the inner conflict we may have over exercising. On the one hand, you want to exercise to improve your health, but on the other, you would just rather be doing something else. This incongruence can be a huge source of conflict in your life and the most effective way to turbocharge your life is to learn to move in harmony with your values.

You will also discover how to improve your environment to help you exercise. This means looking at the parts of your environment that support you in the achievement of your goal (places, people, and things). Which of these things help you to achieve your goals and which are hindering you? For example, you may not currently have anywhere to exercise, there may be people in your life who are not supportive of your desire to optimise your health, or you may not have the equipment you want for your chosen fitness programme.

Finally, we will draw your awareness to your own body, what it is capable of, and what it needs in order to thrive. I will help you set realistic health and fitness goals and develop new habits that will guarantee success. You will start to embrace a new identity and understand how best to get the support and accountability you need for continued success. We are all a work in progress. Caring for your body is a continual process and I am going to help you fall in love with taking the very best care of you.

LONG-TERM SUCCESS

This is not about short-term wins - the bikini body in seven days, or dropping a dress size in two weeks - which invariably bring short-term happiness... and then marches you right back to where you started. This is about long-term, sustainable success for your physical, mental, and emotional wellbeing – body confidence, energy, and joy. You are going to learn how to make exercise happen without overwhelm, so you can thrive. You will let go of perfectionism, guilt, and a fixation with washboard abs, dress sizes, narrower hips, and those pesky scales. While physical changes will happen, they will be a by-product of your new fitness lifestyle, rather than seemingly unattainable goals in themselves. The more you love it and the more you stick with it, the more changes you will see and experience.

But don't worry. This is not going to require an entire overhaul of your lifestyle. These are small tweaks to help fine-tune what you are already doing. It's a different perspective, a mindset shift that will change everything. In order to look and feel different, you need to think differently, allowing your mind and body to work in harmony rather than in constant conflict.

So, let's get started.

CHAPTER SUMMARY

- You're never too old or unfit to move and get fitter.
- Small changes to your mindset and habits can deliver sustainable and significant results.
- Your previous unsuccessful attempts to get fitter may not have been in tune with what makes you tick.
- Understanding yourself and your environment can help you achieve a fitness habit and lifestyle that you love as much as chocolate!

NEXT STEPS

- Grab a notepad and pen to complete the tasks throughout this book. This is a practical learning guide and to make the most out of the experience, you will want to put in the work!
- Get yourself a journal that you can start using while you are reading this book, to help track the shifts in your mindset, your new habits and what you are grateful for. You can take a look at my journal here https://breakingballet.com/journal/, or choose your own. Something that feels luxurious, that will encourage you to curl up on the sofa with a cup of tea and create that time and space just for you.

2

KNOWING YOURSELF

W hen it comes to finding motivation to exercise, one of THE most important factors is to have an in-depth knowledge of yourself and what makes you tick. What motivates you to do things?

I can share all the strategies I use personally to stay consistent with my exercise, but that doesn't mean those strategies are going to work for you.

There is no "one size fits all" approach when it comes to being consistent with exercise. We are all motivated by different factors. If you have been trying to motivate yourself to exercise using the same techniques every time, this will undoubtedly lead to overwhelm, frustration, and negative self-talk when those efforts fail.

WHO AM I?

When we know who we are, what our interests and values are, we can begin to lead a happy and fulfilled life. Self-awareness is the first step to self-improvement. When we can sense and understand our internal world, our mind's pathways are opened.

Focusing on the sensations in our bodies can enhance interoception – the ability to assess and understand information from our body, like hunger, tiredness, pain, and pleasure. When we are able to start linking physical cues (such as a rumbling tummy) with internal states (hunger), we enhance our ability for emotional regulation.

It's about understanding your own needs and desires, understanding your strengths and weaknesses, and being able to accurately assess your emotions.

How well do you think you know the person who is looking back at you in the mirror?

Journal task

Try answering the following questions and see how easily you are able to do so, or whether you are unable to answer all of them.

What do you find meaningful? What are you passionate about?

What are your interests? What are your beliefs? What are your values? What is your purpose? What emotions do you feel most of the time?

Why do you behave the way you do? Who are you underneath the socially constructed self that you have created in order to fit in?

When I first started helping women to achieve their health and fitness goals through exercise, healthy eating, and self-care, I used to get a little frustrated when I could see that these women knew what they needed to do, but were just not doing it.

When I was asked, *"How do you manage to workout on a regular basis?"* it was a simple answer – *"Well, I just do it."* I couldn't understand why other women were not *just* doing it. To me it was simple: you have a goal, you know what is required to achieve it, and you do those things until you get there. I have always operated this way – at school, during my dancing career, at university and law school, and finally, as I rose up the ranks in my legal career. Pick the goal, take action, tick it off the list.

Obviously, there was plenty of hard work involved. I had many challenges along the way and sometimes it involved making life changes that felt uncomfortable. But I had friends who had a similar approach, so most of the time, this way of being felt normal. After all, we only know what we know. It was when I started teaching ballet-inspired fitness classes that I realised the approach I was taking towards achieving my goals (exercise included) was not necessarily always the approach others took. Maybe I was the odd one out? Maybe I needed to loosen up a bit and not be so boring and hell-bent on achieving all the time?

WHAT'S WRONG WITH ME?

I knew the reason exercise wasn't happening for some people wasn't because they were lazy, or didn't want the goal as much as I did, or couldn't work out how to get there. I could see once I had had my own children that this wasn't the case. My children didn't operate in the same way as me either, but some other kids did! Why didn't my kids just do their homework, instead of putting it off and leaving it until the last minute? Why, when I pushed for them to take action towards goals they had set for themselves, did I not only receive resistance, but rebellion? What was I doing wrong?

Of course, it was less to do with my parenting, or teaching skills, and more to do with human nature – the way we operate as individuals and how we process information. I became fascinated with what was driving me, and others like me, to achieve our goals without any real drama. I wanted to know how learning more about our personalities can help us to live the life we want to live, without self-doubt or feeling like the odd one out.

I discovered that knowing how to use your self-awareness to your advantage can help you to achieve anything you want in life:

- If you know your strengths, you can leverage them to live a life that is compatible with your natural talents.
- Knowing your weaknesses can help you choose the right interventions to avoid derailing your progress.
- Knowing your core values means you will make decisions that lead you to a happy and fulfilled life, in alignment with what is important to you.
- Learning to trust your gut instinct will give you self-belief and confidence in your decision-making.
- Taking responsibility for change if things are not going the way you would like them to requires self-awareness to make an honest assessment of what is working and what is not working in your life.

TUNING IN

Improving your fitness requires both mental and physical effort. It's not just about moving your body regularly (if it was, we would all be doing it). An increased self-awareness helps you to understand what has previously held you back from achieving your fitness goals – limiting beliefs that you don't deserve an attractive or healthy body, a fear of injury, or people treating you differently if you make the changes. It also helps to prevent you from injury when you are honest with yourself about what you are currently capable of achieving with your body (the weight you are lifting, or the miles you are running). When you are self-aware you can tune in to how you are feeling on a particular day, so, if necessary, you can adjust the intensity of your workouts to accommodate that.

WHY IS SELF-KNOWLEDGE CRUCIAL?

Self-awareness sits at the centre of emotional intelligence, and viewing your actions from an objective point of view allows you to be fully aware of your behaviours, feelings, and traits. Once you achieve this awareness, you can then take responsibility for your emotions and understand the triggers for them. The more self-awareness you have, the less validation you will seek from others and you will also see others for who they truly are. This helps you to build healthy relationships, which, of course, we know is necessary for our own success.

THE GUILT TRAP

One of the challenges I see women face at this point is a sense of guilt over putting themselves first. Some women see putting their needs above others' as a selfish act. But wanting to achieve something does not make you a selfish person. If you have children, ageing parents, or other loved ones, and you are feeling guilty about time spent exercising instead of spending it with them, try to reframe this. Presumably you want your children to grow up prioritising their health and wellbeing. You want them to be their own person, make choices in life that will make them happy and enable them to live the life they deserve. You also want to be fit and healthy to continue to spend quality time with loved ones or look after those who depend on you. By prioritising your health and fitness, not only are you modelling this behaviour to your children, you are also ensuring you stay fit and strong so you can give your best to others.

Whatever it is you think you "should" be doing instead of focusing on yourself (e.g., career), think about what your hard work and focus is all for. Don't you owe it to yourself to look after your body and mind so that you can be as strong and able as possible, to enjoy life to the full as you get older and when you retire?

You are responsible for taking action to achieve your health and fitness goals. It is work you will need to do. This means you need to be your best self, which can only be achieved through self-awareness.

GAINING SELF-AWARENESS

There are many ways to gain more self-awareness. At first it can all seem a bit "woo". You have lived with yourself all your life so surely you know who you are, right?! So, what are you supposed to do to *get to know yourself*? Well, it's not too dissimilar to getting to know somebody else. It's a case of sitting and listening to your thoughts, dreams, and feelings about your life.

There are many different exercises you can do to gain self-awareness. Here are a few examples to get you started:

- Start to question your negative thought patterns. If you are an "all or nothing" person and your actions don't live up to your perfectionism ideals, you have a tendency to see yourself as a total failure. You might dwell on the one negative comment someone made about you rather than the 26 positive ones you heard that week. You may also be prone to discounting positive experiences because for some reason they "don't count". By accepting these thoughts as true, it is distorting your perception of reality. Instead, become aware of these thought patterns. Journal on them and start to replace them with more positive thoughts that more accurately reflect your reality.

- Write down your strengths and weaknesses. What are you good at and what do people compliment you on? When you have achieved success in life, what strengths did you use to achieve that success? As for your weaknesses, what do you avoid doing? When you have experienced failure in life, what actions or behaviours led to that failure? Once you have the answers to these questions, it will enable you to focus on the strengths and manage the weaknesses when it comes to exercising.

- Increasing your physical awareness helps you to gain a strong sense of what is happening in your body at any given moment. Yoga and ballet are wonderful in-the-moment activities and will help connect your mind and body. The mind-body connection means that your thoughts, feelings, and beliefs can positively, or negatively, affect your biological functioning. In other words, your mind can affect how healthy your body is. On the other hand, what you do with your physical body (what you eat, how much you exercise, even your posture) can impact your mental state - again, positively or negatively.

- Ask trusted friends for their input. This can feel like an awkward exercise for some, but it is very powerful. Ask them for feedback on your personality – positive and negative. This will help you to gain a better understanding of how you are perceived by others.
- Listen to your self-talk. Observe the things you say to yourself each day and write them down, word for word. When you look back over your notes you will start to see a pattern emerging and this will give you greater insight into how you speak to yourself.
- Create a vision board and fill it with everything you want to be, do, and have in life. These can be short, medium, and long-term goals. It can be made up of images, photos, words, or a mixture of all three. It is a visual representation of your bucket list. Forget how you are going to achieve any of these things. Just have a clear vision of what they are for now. Knowing what you really want out of life will help you become more self-aware. It will also help you discover your personal reason for exercising, which we will come to later. It's not necessarily what you think it is!
- Take a personality test. I have done many of these over the years, including Myers Briggs. I also did psychometric testing before changing my career and found it really helpful to focus on where my passion lies. However, when I came across Gretchen Rubin's "The Four Tendencies" framework, it finally all made total sense. Not only could I identify my tendencies and my behaviours clearly, I could also identify the tendencies of friends, my husband, my children and

my clients. When it comes to discovering what motivates you, it is an incredible tool to truly understand why you do what you do and what strategies you can put in place to achieve your fitness goals.

THE FOUR TENDENCIES

Of course, no single system can capture human nature in all its depth and variety, but The Four Tendencies looks at just one aspect of a person's character – why we act and why we don't act – so it is the most relevant system for the purposes of looking at your motivation to exercise. The Four Tendencies is a spotlight to help us tweak situations to boost our chances of success, not a box with a label we are putting ourselves in.

In her book, "The Four Tendencies", Rubin invites you to ask yourself the simple question *"How do I respond to expectations?"* Based on your answer to this question you will fit into one of four tendencies:

1. Upholder
2. Questioner
3. Obliger
4. Rebel.

Your Tendency shapes your behaviour, and understanding your Tendency helps you to make better decisions, stick to your habits, be more productive, reduce stress, and communicate more effectively with others. Most importantly for the purposes of this book, it can also help you to find the best strategies to motivate yourself to move. Let's take a look at each Tendency. See if you can identify yourself in any of these descriptions.

Upholder

The upholder meets both outer and inner expectations. Discipline is their freedom and they love schedules and routines. They find it easy to decide to act and follow through. They can more easily form habits than the other tendencies and don't depend on others to motivate them. They are completely independent. As a result, they are less prone to resentment and burnout. They value self-mastery and performance and so, take satisfaction and enjoyment from upholding their habits (exercise, healthy eating, quality sleep etc.). Letting themselves off the hook is not really an option and can often make them feel worse. Upholders make up only 19% of the population, making them one of the smaller groups behind Rebels (17%).

Questioner

For the Questioner, justification leads to motivation. They meet only inner expectations. To take action, they need to gather their own facts, decide for themselves, and act with good reason. They will only meet expectations if they consider them efficient and reasonable. For example, if a questioner wants to get fit, they will need to be convinced that a particular form of exercise is right, by doing copious amounts of research, weighing up all the options and deciding it is the most productive way to get fit. They are prepared to ignore other people's rules or expectations and are able to follow through on their plans without much difficulty.

The downside is they sometimes suffer from analysis paralysis and can find loopholes if they want to avoid doing a particular habit. If they don't agree with an outer expectation (someone suggesting they do something), they feel entitled to dismiss it. Questioners are the second largest group of the four tendencies (behind Obligers) at 24%.

Obliger

Obligers readily meet outer expectations, but resist inner expectations. No matter how much they want to meet inner expectations, they often fail. The only way they seem to be able to meet their inner expectations is by creating outer accountability. This is the crucial part for them in achieving their goals. Knowing the type of outer accountability that works for them is the secret to their success.

Obligers are the largest group in the tendencies framework (41%) and have the most to gain from learning about their tendency. They feel a sense of obligation to others and so, are more likely to succeed if they frame a goal as a benefit to others instead of as a personal value. They can meet expectations if they are tied to their duty of being a good role model. Because of their people-pleasing nature, they are susceptible to burnout.

Rebel

Rebels resist meeting inner and outer expectations. They hate being told what to do, even if they are telling themselves what to do! They want to take action based on a sense of freedom, choice, and self-expression, and place a high value on being true to themselves. They want to do things their own way and resist anything that they perceive to be an attempt at control.

They resist committing to a schedule, or doing boring tasks, unless they can see the very real benefits of doing so. Rebels respond best to a pattern of information, consequences, and choice. We have to give them the information they need to make an informed decision, explain the likely consequences of their actions and then let them make the choice. Rebels account for just 17% of the population.

Can you see yourself in one of these Tendencies?

When I discovered I'm an Upholder, my life finally all made total sense. As a child, I would spend the summer holidays working on projects to keep myself occupied and in a routine. I set rules around when I would work, what the end product would look like and I didn't care if anyone even looked at it. My brother (who as a child came out in a rash if he needed to read, or do anything that might look like school work) thought I was weird. Is being an Upholder the most glamorous, edgy, or interesting quality? No. Is it any surprise that I went on to become a lawyer and then an entrepreneur? No. But it's who I am. And it took me years to realise that not everyone else is like this, and even longer to accept that this is who I am and it's ok. But it has been life-changing in so many ways.

So which Tendency are you?

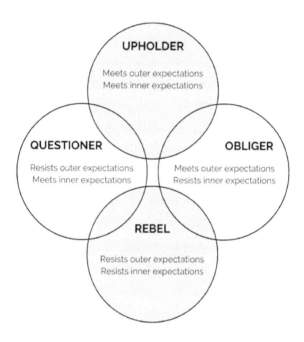

As you can see from the above image, there can be some overlap with the Tendencies and a particular Tendency can "tip" in the direction of one of the overlapping Tendencies. For example, an Upholder/Obliger tips towards responding to outer expectations.

At the end of this chapter, you will take the Four Tendencies quiz and learn which Tendency you are. I have applied the Four Tendencies framework throughout this book to help you answer the question, *"How do I make exercise happen?"* This will enable you to identify the right personal strategies to help motivate you and inspire you towards living a healthier and more active life. For example, if you are an Obliger, you are going to be far more likely to exercise consistently if there is an expectation from someone else that you will do it. So, in this case, having an accountability partner, or a group of women to support you, is vital. On the other hand, if you are an Upholder, you are better able to set your own expectations of yourself and stick to them. So, next time you are giving yourself a hard time for skipping your workout, stop. Remember, that it might just be that you are not using the right strategies to help motivate you. What is working for your friend is not necessarily going to work for you. But we are going to figure all this out together.

CHAPTER SUMMARY

- There is no "one size fits all" solution to exercise and fitness.
- A greater self-awareness is key to understanding the fitness regime that will work for you and be sustainable in the long-term.
- It's about finding a regime that complements your strengths and is in tune with your core values.
- You are responsible for your health and fitness and for being a role model for your children.
- Understanding yourself is not as simple as it sounds. We are not in the habit of doing it. You need to take time to listen to your thoughts, dreams and feelings.

- Use the techniques in this book to identify your Tendency, to help you better understand what will motivate you to exercise.

NEXT STEPS:

- Take The Four Tendencies quiz. Go to https://quiz.gretchenrubin.com/four-tendencies-quiz/ and complete the quiz. It will only take you around 10 minutes.
- Write down 3 characteristics of your Tendency that you can most relate to in the table below.

TENDENCY	CHARACTERISTICS
Upholder	1. 2. 3.
Questioner	1. 2. 3.
Obliger	1. 2. 3.
Rebel	1. 2. 3.

- Write down your strengths and weaknesses. Ask trusted friends for their input.

- Listen to your self-talk. Observe the things you say to yourself each day and write them down, word for word.
- Create a vision board and fill it with everything you want to be, do and have in life. These can be short, medium and long-term goals. It can be made up of images, photos, words or a mixture of all three.

3

MOTIVATION TO MOVE

> "Avoiding death isn't a big enough incentive. The only reliable motivation to exercise is vanity."[1]

I s this true, or has this been true, for you? It's certainly a thought-provoking statement.

As a child, I never thought about exercise as something people did to stay healthy, or to change, or maintain their appearance. I don't remember being taught this at school, or my parents telling me I needed to get out of the house and move my body (they weren't trying to get us off screens then!). But I was brought up in a house where movement was normal. My mum played squash weekly, went to yoga and "Pop-mobility", played in the occasional tennis match and walked the dogs daily. My dad (who had me when he was 50 years old) was less active in his later years, but had been a cross-country runner in his youth. He taught us to swim and was an avid follower of sports. He was our biggest cheerleader.

My brother excelled at all sports, particularly rugby (we grew up in Wales). I also loved sport, but in my teenage years that took a back seat when the focus became very much on my dancing.

So in our house, movement was part of our lifestyle and it was fun. It meant we got to spend time with our friends and family (I often went to exercise classes with my mum, wearing some very special leotard combinations), enjoyed being part of a team, or achieving the next grade in dance. We were highly competitive (both with ourselves and others) and needed no encouragement to train, practice, focus and improve our performance.

I am acutely aware that not everyone has the same experience growing up. I have friends who didn't have active parents and did not take part in sports as a child for multiple different reasons, and yes, this can have an impact on how you view exercising as an adult (which we will look at in Chapter 4).

BUT... my lifestyle completely changed when I went to University. I stopped dancing. I didn't join any sports clubs, other than the netball team on a fairly irregular basis, and went to a grand total of two exercise classes during my three-year degree. Why? I was finding enjoyment elsewhere. I had moved away from home for the first time, had the freedom to do whatever I wanted and was fully committed to studying in-between having (too much) fun. I don't remember it ever entering my mind to "exercise". None of my friends were exercising, or taking part in any sports clubs. We were having the time of our lives doing other things, like meeting new friends, discovering new bars, drinking too much alcohol, and getting to grips with how to cook meals and clean our clothes.

Looking back now, I find this baffling. I loved movement and yet I spent a significant proportion of my life not doing any at all. There was no necessity for exercise. I wasn't motivated to do it any more, despite having the skills and capabilities and having grown up in an environment that fully supported it. I would have still enjoyed it if I had taken part, but it just wasn't on my radar. I no longer had a *reason* to move my body.

Given you are reading this book, I know that, at this stage in your life, you have a reason to move your body. So what is motivation and how do we harness it to help us move?

WHAT IS MOTIVATION?

"Motivation" = a reason for acting in a particular way.

Motivation is the driving force behind human behaviour. It helps to direct and maintain our goal-oriented actions. Motivation is a condition inside us that desires a change, either for ourselves, or our environment.

For the purposes of exercise, it's helpful to see your motivation in two parts:

1. *Why* you exercise; and

2. The sorts of things that will keep you going, even when it gets tough.

This book will share lots of strategies that help to motivate you to keep exercising, but understanding why you are starting in the first place is crucial, especially when it comes to helping you set your goals and achieve them, as we discuss in Chapter 6.

YOUR WHY

I have been asked so many times how long it takes to create a habit. People still believe that repetition creates habits - if they can stick it out for X number of days, they will have achieved their goal. Yes, repetition and frequency go some way towards creating habits that will lead you towards your goal, but habits tend to form much more quickly if you have a strong positive emotion connected to the behaviour.[2] We will look at this shortly, but it's worth keeping in mind when you are setting what I call your "destination goal" – your one big fitness goal.

Whilst your destination goal can seem like the holy grail, let's look at the meaning behind your goal because, as we now know, it's how we stay motivated with our exercise. Why do you want to achieve your destination goal? When you have the answer, continue to drill down and ask why for each answer you give. Let's use Anna as an example:

Me: What's your goal?
Anna: To lose three stone.

Me: Why?

Anna: So I can fit into my jeans again.

Me: Why is that important?

Anna: Because I can't get into them at the moment and it makes me feel miserable.

Me: How will you feel when you do fit into them?

Anna: Much more confident!

Me: Why is that important?

Anna: My confidence is low. If it improves, I will be able to maintain some healthy boundaries around my habits.

Me: What will that mean for you?

Anna: That I can stand up for myself and feel proud of my achievements. Then maybe I will be able to assert myself more at work…

And so it goes on. You get the picture. The weight loss goal is much more than a weight loss goal. It is a goal that will also help improve Anna's mental and emotional wellbeing, at the same time as experiencing physical changes that will inevitably benefit her health. This shifts the focus from the ultimate goal, to the importance of sticking to your behaviours (even on bad or busy days when you don't want to). You already do this each day in other areas of your life. You may go to a job that you don't like (or even hate). Why? Because it's important. Maybe it's paying the mortgage, or for the annual holidays. Something is more important to you than the time it takes to do a job that you don't even like.

My "why" is future-proofing my body and mind so I'm an active woman in my 70s and 80s, playing with my grandchildren and travelling the world. Of course, when I was younger, my reasons for exercising were very much entangled with body image and living up to certain body standards. Honestly, it is still important for me to feel comfortable in my clothes. Part of my identity is wrapped up in being slim and toned, so it would be uncomfortable for me to put on weight or feel like I was losing strength. But this is not the ONLY thing that drives my exercise.

Painting a picture

To help you gain clarity around your why, try painting as clear a picture as possible in response to the following question: *Imagine yourself as a child looking through a window into your work, or home life twelve months from now. They have come to see what it will be like as an adult. What would you like them to see you doing? What sort of scene would make them feel proud of their adult self and reassure them that when it comes to the habits you have control over, everything is great?*

You can repeat this exercise but rather than imagining yourself as a child, instead imagine yourself as a 75-year-old woman, looking back at your life twelve months from now. Is she proud of what she sees and grateful for the effort you are putting in now?

EXAMPLES OF WHAT YOUR WHY MIGHT LOOK LIKE
"I want to live a long, happy life, free from pain"
"I want to be a role model for my children, to ensure they prioritise their health in adulthood"
"I want to be around to play with my grandchildren"
"I want to have energy to continue doing the work I love"
"I want to feel body confident so I can live life to the full"

TYPES OF MOTIVATION

Typically, there are two types of motivation: extrinsic and intrinsic.

1. Extrinsic motivations arise from outside the individual, like winning a trophy, gaining recognition from others, receiving money, or pressures arising out of the social context of our environment.
2. Intrinsic motivations arise from inside the individual and comprise their needs, cognitions, and emotions, like personal gratification from completing a workout.

These intrinsic and extrinsic motivations are the same as the inner and outer expectations Rubin talks about in The Four Tendencies.

While I was dancing as a child, I was mostly intrinsically motivated. I had a strong desire for personal achievement and improvement and wanted to prove to myself that I could achieve the top grades, master the next challenging pirouette sequence or pointe work routine. However, there was also a part of me that wanted to please my teacher, see how proud my parents were and outperform other students (I'm still competitive). I was curious as to whether my talent would hold up against other students across the country, auditioning for ballet school, or whether I was good, but not particularly special. These extrinsic motivations were the rewards I got at the end of all my hard work. I appreciated external praise, as I wasn't great at celebrating my own wins.

I later realised that I also had a need to belong as a child. I wanted to fit in and be liked. I didn't ever feel like I belonged at school and dance provided me with a safe haven. Dancing meant I was together with other girls who understood how dance made me feel. Their enjoyment was my enjoyment. We were all good at different aspects of our dancing and we shared tips and supported each other. It felt like a team, a family. This made me want to show up early on a Saturday morning and limber up with my friends before our teacher arrived for the day. It made me want to spend the vast majority of my time outside of school in a dance studio, choreographing and experimenting with different pieces of music.

To gain a better understanding of your personal motivation, now is a good time to take a look at how you have been motivated to move in the past. Did your strategy work? If not, how can you best change your approach going forward?

WHAT HAS MOTIVATED YOU IN THE PAST?

Motivating yourself to exercise is usually done in one of two ways:

1. Creating anxiety, or
2. Imagining a positive experience.

When you motivate yourself through anxiety, you are saying things like *"If I don't exercise, I'll put on weight"*, or *"I won't fit into my new dress"*. In our work lives we motivate ourselves with deadlines, which create enough anxiety (usually) to motivate us to get the job done. It creates adrenaline, which is what gets us moving.

On the flip side, you can change your strategy by creating a positive experience. You can tell yourself you are looking forward to moving, or seeing your friend for a walk. You can track your progress and be proud of how hard you are working. You can focus on completing your workout and how amazing you will feel at the end.

Journal task

Take a moment now to reflect on your life and the times where you have succeeded in achieving a particular goal (any goal, not just a fitness related goal).

- What drove you to achieve that goal?
- Did other people play a part in that?

- What was the reward at the end and what did that mean to you?
- Ask yourself why you put in the effort and what was important to you about achieving your goal. Was it a drive, or a need?

Now, think about a time you started a new exercise programme.

- Was it for fun, to create a personal challenge, for health benefits, for an emotional kick, to accomplish a goal, to improve your mood, or to spend time with friends?
- Were you forced to do it?
- Did you do it to alleviate guilt, or relieve stress and anxiety?
- Or, did you do it because you felt body shamed in some way and wanted to change your appearance?

As you gain a deeper understanding throughout this book about what motivates you, this will help you to take action to move your body, engage in health-oriented behaviours, avoid unhealthy behaviours, and feel happier and more in control of your life. Knowing what motivates you improves your efficiency as you work towards your goals.

HOW YOU SABOTAGE YOUR MOTIVATION

Your motivation, or willpower, will of course have ups and downs. We are very adept at avoiding exercise when we want to.

Whether this is due to perfectionism, comparison with others, unrealistic expectations, imposter syndrome, or something completely different, we can easily find an excuse to sabotage our goals.

Chapter 4 in this book will help you to become more aware of these self-sabotaging patterns and arm you with strategies to keep moving forward despite the pull to take the path of least resistance and avoid exercise altogether.

For now, here are some common pitfalls you can start to observe straight away:

Quick fixes

"All or nothing" thinking doesn't work. If you can't fix something straight away, or if you can't have it all at once, it's easy to feel unmotivated. Remind yourself that your health and fitness goals take time and effort.

One size fits all

Just because a particular fitness regime, or healthy eating programme is working for your friend, doesn't mean it's going to work for you. If something isn't helping you to reach your goal, or is making you feel unmotivated, look for something else that works better for you.

The little voice

The little voice in your head is very powerful when it comes to helping you to avoid exercise. Have you ever had the following thoughts, or said these words (or similar) out loud?

"I'm not motivated"

"I don't have any energy"

"I don't have enough time"

"I'm not consistent and quit when life gets in the way"

"I'm overwhelmed and don't know where to start"

"I would prefer not to".

These are the most common excuses I hear from women not working out regularly. But is it a lack of motivation that is the real problem?

IS IT REALLY A LACK OF MOTIVATION?

"Exercise" = *optional* physical activity for the sake of health and fitness.

It's the word *"optional"* that is the issue here. Voluntary physical exercise is not natural. We never evolved to exercise. Our hunter-gatherer ancestors didn't run, or walk for miles for the sake of their health. They had to be physically active for hours each day to get enough food and stay safe.

So you see, it's not your fault if you are currently avoiding exercise!

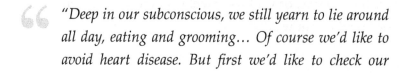
"Deep in our subconscious, we still yearn to lie around all day, eating and grooming... Of course we'd like to avoid heart disease. But first we'd like to check our

phones. Maybe get a snack. Relax a little. If exercise isn't going to make me look hot, it can wait".[3]

We know that physical activity is vital to help slow ageing and promote fitness and health. But as we are no longer engaging in physical labour as our ancestors did, it means we must now exercise to maintain our health. That said, we know it's not as simple as putting on your trainers and hoping your legs will carry you out of the front door. It takes a little re-wiring.

In fact, exercise seems to have become a source of anxiety and confusion for many of us, because even though we all know it is good for our health, we struggle to exercise enough, to work out safely, or even to find the joy in it. This is because our minds never evolved to get us moving unless it is *necessary, enjoyable,* or in some other way *rewarding.*[4]

How to make exercise necessary

If you are not overweight or suffering from a medical condition, you may not see the *need* to move your body right now. If you have little, or no, need for achievement, you may experience a negative effect, such as anxiety, shame, and embarrassment while engaging in that challenging task and will avoid, or procrastinate as a result. Part of the problem is the distinction between *"should"* and *"need"*. *"I should lose weight to be more attractive."* This type of thinking may induce feelings of guilt or shame, or lead us to feel frustration, anger, or bitterness. So what can we do?

- Focus on exercising to future-proof your body, decreasing your risk of illnesses that tend to surface in later life.
- Focus on your *'why'*: this could be for longevity, being able to play with your children/grandchildren, to avoid injury, or to maintain your weight as you age.
- Find compassionate help. People saying *"just do it"* is not helpful. Find people who will encourage and support you through the ups and downs. Whether that's family, a personal trainer, or even a friend who you can exercise with.
- Make it simple and achievable. Focus on short, effective workouts that you can do every day, and diarise them to track your progress.
- Make yourself accountable. Schedule in exercise with a friend, join a group or sign up for a race so that you can feel more committed and will be responsible for showing up regularly.

We will be looking in more detail at some of these different strategies in later chapters and how some may be more effective than others, depending on your Tendency.

How to make exercise enjoyable

Do you remember watching Back to the Future 3?

Doc: And in the future, we don't need horses. We have motorised carriages called automobiles.

Saloon Old Timer: If everybody's got one of these auto-whatsits, does anybody walk or run anymore?

Doc: Of course we run. But for recreation. For fun.

Saloon Old Time: Run for fun? What the hell kind of fun is that?

Even if you find a form of exercise enjoyable, it is not always going to be fun. You might start off full of enthusiasm and relief at finding a form of exercise you actually don't hate, but you will still have bad or busy days, when all you want to do is crash on the sofa with a glass of wine and a bar of chocolate and watch the latest Netflix series. So how do we make exercise more enjoyable?

- Make it sociable. Busy people can find time to do things they enjoy, so find your tribe and have some fun.
- Focus on how good you feel after exercising; this will help to motivate you next time around.
- Choose exercise you enjoy, or dislike the least! There is no point choosing to run if you hate running (although you can learn to love an exercise you initially hate). Instead, start with something enjoyable and then apply the strategies in this book to help you sustain the habit.
- Entertain yourself while working out by listening to your favourite music or podcast.

How to reward yourself

Rewarding yourself immediately after exercise is proven to be one of the most powerful ways of maintaining the habit by helping to rewire your brain. We will discuss this in more depth in Chapter 7.

HOW TO MOTIVATE YOURSELF ACCORDING TO YOUR TENDENCY

Understanding your unique personality and how you operate is key to identifying your motivation when it comes to exercise. The table below shows how you are likely to be motivated, according to your Tendency.

TENDENCY	MOTIVATION	TAKEAWAY
Upholder	• If you decide to start exercising you will. Even if other people don't care. • You don't need others to motivate you. • You meet BOTH inner and outer expectations. • Your determination to meet inner expectations will be improved if you can see that strengthening yourself will help you meet others' expectations.	Make a decision to start exercising.
Questioner	• You are motivated by reason, logic and fairness. • You need to decide for yourself whether a particular form of exercise is a good idea. It needs to have a sound purpose. • If you see exercise as worthwhile, you'll stick to it.	Find a purpose for your exercise.
Obliger	• You have a need to be a good role model. • You find it difficult to exercise for your benefit only. • You need external accountability to maintain an exercise regime.	See exercise as something you do to be a good role model to others.
Rebel	• You resist rules around exercise, especially if there's an expectation you are to do it regularly. • You can only embrace an exercise regime if you can tie the exercise to your own decision-making. • You can reframe how you view exercise and end up with a regular routine by taking it one day at a time, deciding to do it "this time".	Exercise has to be your choice. I can't tell you what to do!

REFRAMING THE WAY YOU VIEW EXERCISE

Taking small steps to reframe the way you think about exercise is key to finding it a source of pleasure and health, rather than a cause of discomfort, guilt and shame.

If you are not currently prioritising your health and fitness, and this is something you WANT to do, the chances are you are telling yourself you are hopeless, lazy, lacking in willpower, or something similar. This negative self-talk serves no purpose other than to make you feel crap about yourself. It doesn't spur you on to make the necessary changes. How can you start exercising if you believe you are lazy? How will you focus on your healthy eating if you think you are hopeless? Lazy, hopeless people don't make a success of themselves. But you can.

It is human nature to want to take the path of least resistance. To rest and have food delivered to the door rather than plan, shop, cook, and wash up. It is human nature to drive a car rather than walk, park nearer to the supermarket doors, or stay under the duvet on a cold morning.

But none of this is going to lead you towards lifelong health and happiness. You are more than capable of shifting those unwanted pounds, feeling comfortable in your clothes and looking and feeling the best you have in years.

CHAPTER SUMMARY

- Exercise is self-care. It can improve your physical condition, but also the way you feel. But voluntary exercise is not natural - we evolved to move when it's necessary, enjoyable, or rewarding in some other way.
- You need to understand what will motivate you to exercise - what is your reason? There's no right or wrong answer.

- Knowing what has successfully motivated you in other contexts will help you develop a method to improve your efficiency in achieving your fitness goals.

NEXT STEPS:

1. IDENTIFY YOUR "WHY"

Think about why you want to exercise. You can use the example table earlier in this chapter to help, but it's a very personal process. There are no right or wrong reasons for exercise. Write your list of reasons in the table below.

MY REASONS FOR EXERCISING

2. LACK OF CONFIDENCE

Lack of confidence in your ability to motivate yourself to exercise is a barrier to exercising. Sometimes you can feel like it's not reasonable to feel confident when your mind is telling you that you are hopeless, lazy, and have no willpower. But we can start to rewire your brain a little here by finding your "Greatest Hits".

1. Think of a situation where you had full confidence and motivation to complete a task, or goal. Where you knew exactly how to manage whatever it was that could arise. Your list above may help you here. Try to place yourself back into that very situation. Rerun in your mind the movie of that experience as slowly as you can. Let go of any judgement you may have around the strategies you used.

2. Notice what comes up for you when you think of that experience. Do you see a picture? Do you hear anything? What feelings come up and where in your body?

3. Develop a list of these experiences and try to be "in" the movie and feel how wonderful you felt.

Making a list of your motivators and recalling your Greatest Hits will not only change your thought processes, but will also provide a useful evidence log of all the times you have been successful in motivating yourself to complete a task. When in doubt, you can refer back to these lists to remind yourself that you are more than capable of motivating yourself to take action.

EXAMPLE "GREATEST HITS"
"I made a presentation at work to all my colleagues. I felt nervous but I was determined to perform well. I was well prepared and got great feedback - someone told me it was one of the best sessions they had attended at work. I was so proud of myself. During the presentation, I managed to relax and felt on top of the world. I answered questions confidently and realised I really know my stuff! It was a feeling of excitement moving through my body, and I was full of energy. The room was quiet and I had captured everyone's attention."

BELIEFS SHAPE YOUR REALITY

Charlotte wanted to lose some vanity pounds and start really prioritising her health and wellbeing. She was quite happy with her eating habits but was frustrated at her perceived inability to exercise regularly. She was exercising now and again, but was finding excuses not to do so and when she did exercise, she was not really pushing herself very hard. She easily gave up when things became a little uncomfortable.

Throughout her childhood, Charlotte believed she was weak and in poor health. As a child, she had a medical issue with one of her eyes and her mother was fearful that if she over exerted herself, the eye condition would deteriorate. So her mother wrote a letter to the school excusing Charlotte from taking part in PE lessons in case it exacerbated her eye condition. Charlotte was signed off PE for most of her school life.

Her parents told her that she was delicate and needed to be careful with her body.

Despite not experiencing any issues with her eyes in adulthood, Charlotte continued to believe this narrative. That she needed to take great care when it came to exercising. As a result, she started to avoid exercise, even when she knew it was good for her physical, mental and emotional health. Exercise was something she recommended to her own clients in her executive coaching business, but she was unable to really push her fitness beyond walking in the mountains, and even that provided some level of anxiety.

When we delved a little deeper into the impact that was having on her now, we discovered that she had a deep-rooted fear of pain, or discomfort, when exercising. She really didn't feel comfortable exercising and it caused her anxiety. When she started to feel her heart rate increase, or her breath becoming more laboured, or her muscles start to ache, she would seize up and sometimes break down in tears. There was no medical reason, or indication, preventing her from exercising.

Growing up, Alicia, 36, a mum of two young boys, suffered from asthma. She disliked PE lessons at school and avoided joining in with sporting activities. This was in part because she was not selected by her peers to join their team and because she felt she didn't have the stamina to join in. As an adult, Alicia struggled to believe she had the right to take care of herself over and above anyone else. She had developed a fear of cardiovascular exercise, including running, so she avoided it. One of her goals was to lose weight, but this was proving a challenge as she was rarely increasing her heart rate during exercise. She still believed she was the wheezy kid at school that was no good at sport. This old belief was preventing her from taking part in more vigorous physical activity.

At school, Deb was uncoordinated and was never picked for school teams. Teachers commented on how clumsy she was and she felt like the butt of everyone's jokes. This meant that after leaving school, Deb didn't exercise for years, until she hit her 40s. At this stage she started to experience aches and pains in her body and after much deliberation, she decided to attend a yoga class. This was the key to unlocking her confidence with movement. She had discovered in adulthood that she had Dyspraxia (a condition affecting physical co-ordination), which explained her lack of co-ordination as a child. It wasn't her fault. Yes, she was a bit clumsy but there was a reason for it. Once she had grown in confidence, she was able to join my BBackstage community, which increased her confidence even further, allowing her subsequently to start running.

You can see from these three examples, that our beliefs around exercise and our attachment to those beliefs, can prevent us from living our lives to the full until we are able to identify these beliefs for what they are: limiting and, in some cases, completely unfounded.

WHAT IS A BELIEF?

A belief is something you consider to be a fact. These "truths" are used to help us navigate the world and also to keep us safe. This is why we hold on to and guard beliefs that are formed in childhood. Beliefs become our subconscious autopilot. They become ingrained and we assume they are facts, whether they are true or not. Our beliefs determine whether we see something as good or bad, desirable or undesirable, achievable or unachievable.

HOW ARE YOUR BELIEFS FORMED?

As you can see from the above examples, most of our core beliefs are formed in childhood. These beliefs are usually formed in two ways:

1. By our experiences; and
2. By accepting what others tell us to be true.

This can be by a parent, teacher, or peers at school. We believe our parents when they tell us about Santa Claus and the Tooth Fairy. We are later influenced by our changing social environment. When we accept something to be a fact, it is stored in our subconscious mind. Our subconscious mind doesn't deal with true or false, it just stores the fact to "help" us later on.

You're on autopilot

Our subconscious mind acts as our autopilot, making our life easier, much like once you have learned to drive a car (using the brakes, clutch, gears etc.), it all starts to feel natural. This can also be helpful when you are driving home from work on the usual route. You don't have to make many conscious decisions. Your subconscious knows exactly where to go and when to turn left or right when you reach a familiar junction. The journey is easy. Your beliefs are shaping your thoughts and responses. Some of these beliefs serve you well and keep you out of danger, but some, which are not based on fact, serve to hold you back.

How you think, act and feel is based on your beliefs. Limiting or negative beliefs prevent you from leading a full and fulfilled life and cause you to experience negative thoughts and emotions. Conversely, positive beliefs allow you to believe in yourself, be more resilient, and create positive emotions.

Some people are not aware of their beliefs and how they are dictating their reality. As soon as you take the time to analyse your beliefs, you can begin to unlock a strategy to thrive. Now imagine how you would think, feel and act based on one of the following examples of limiting beliefs, or negative thinking around exercise:

EXAMPLES OF LIMITING BELIEFS
"I don't have time to exercise because I need to get the laundry on." (procrastination)
"Everyone else at the gym is lifting heavy weights, so I think I should be doing that too." (conformity / social pressure)
"What if I don't manage to do an hour's workout 3 times this week? And how am I going to fit in cardio, strength training and stretching each week? What if I don't see results in 2 weeks?" (overthinking)
"I don't think I will go to that class tonight. I will make a fool of myself. I'm so uncoordinated." (anxiety)
"I have no idea what I'm doing. Why did I even come here? Who do I think I am?" (imposter syndrome)

The good news is, once you break emotional ties from the past, there will no longer be any pull to cause you to return to the same automatic patterns of your old self.

WHAT ARE YOUR CURRENT EXERCISE BEHAVIOURS?

You are not your behaviour. You have the freedom to choose how you behave in accordance with your identity, or the identity you want to reinforce. We all have bad days and can easily slip back into our old way of being, but it's now time to take responsibility for changing this.

The first step is awareness. See if you can identify yourself in any of these self-sabotaging exercise behavioural patterns.[1]

Quitter: Quitters tend to be out of touch with themselves, their emotions, and others around them. Quitters hide out in the shadows, away from the group. They are easily distracted, do not commit, believe the effort of exercise is not worth the reward, and talk themselves out of what they most desire.

Bull in a China Shop: The Bull keeps on looking for fitness breakthroughs, but is never truly transformed because she is not celebrating her own results and what is important to her in her life now! Bulls have a hard time being satisfied with themselves. They think being the strongest and showing it off is the only way to win. They also seek approval from being the top dog and will do anything to get there.

Ostrich: The Ostrich is not sure she has found the right exercise regime that will give her results/make a real difference, so she buries her head in the sand and grows increasingly demotivated. She refuses to deal with this challenging situation or seek help, choosing instead to continue in the same old pattern.

Run-a-Way: The Run-a-way is stuck in a place of Busy-ness instead of taking the time to focus on what is most important in the Busi-ness of her life. She takes massive action without a clear focus on the long term outcomes. She engages in what she knows she can do easily and effortlessly in the short term and never takes on the real problems she is facing.

Victim: The Victim plays the blame game, noticeable by a very low tolerance for handling the problems and challenges in life. She is reluctant to take responsibility, pushing it off on to others instead. She often feels she is a "victim of circumstance" and doesn't believe she has any control over the circumstances she finds herself in.

Wizard of Oz: The Wizard of Oz believes that there is reward without action. She believes in the "Secret" and the "Law of Attraction". If she can just believe with enough will power, things will happen. She believes in shaping the future, but she just "hopes" it will become so. She believes the answer is out there, somewhere over the rainbow, and somehow, some way, it is going to happen.

Worry Wart: Fear takes over the worry wart. She focuses most of her energy on what may happen, instead of looking at what she wants to make happen. Fear means a person is not prepared for something they perceive may happen in the future. Many times there is too much focus on what they "don't" want to happen.

Actor: the actor works to show that everything is always perfect in their world. For them, it is a challenge to face the truth and live in a way that others may not approve. Actors do not have their own opinions and are always agreeable to what others do. They have to keep up with the Jones' and will do anything to put on a good show for others.

Do you see yourself anywhere here? You may be across more than one pattern. Or, you may have been one in the past and now find you have moved to another. Or, you may have created your own behavioural pattern! Are you able to see how you may have got here? Were there experiences in your life that led you to believe certain things to be true that have caused you to behave this way on repeat? How does this make you feel? What is important is that you can identify your behavioural pattern in relation to exercise. One of the most common ways women avoid exercising is through procrastination. If you do this, you may have related to the Quitter above!

THE PROCRASTINATION TRAP

If you find yourself delaying or postponing your exercise, you are procrastinating. Most busy women procrastinate. We always have more on our to-do list than can get done. And inaction, in the form of procrastination, feels safe and comfortable. If you examine anything in your life that you are putting off, the likelihood is it is because your brain is trying to protect you. It's like a helicopter parent, hovering around, warning you not to do things "just in case". You may be starting to feel like you have lost control of your mind (as well as your motivation to exercise), but this is because the brain is stuck in survival mode. This feeling of being stuck, or procrastinating, is just another behaviour - just not a particularly helpful one. So, what do you do? You have to interrupt these old self-sabotaging patterns and consciously create new neural pathways. If your thoughts and emotions repeat themselves from day to day, you will end up creating the same situations, resulting in the same emotions, and the same thoughts, and, guess what? More procrastinating.

WHAT BELIEFS HAVE YOU ALREADY CREATED?

To gain a better understanding of who you are and how you want to empower your life, you need to look at what you have already created. This is where self-awareness comes in again.

Look at your beliefs about life, yourself and others. You are what you are, you are where you are, and you are who you are because of what you believe about yourself. Whether you are aware of them or not, they still affect your life. You may be reading this book because the strategies you have used in the past to motivate yourself to exercise have not worked. Hopefully, now you are beginning to see that everything in your life is a reflection of your inner beliefs. You can look at your experiences to see what you believe in. Similarly, the people around you are a reflection of what you believe about yourself. If you often go along with what others want to do, you may not be valuing your own opinion. You can sabotage your own health goals if you harbour unconscious beliefs that you do not deserve to achieve them.

What we want in life can differ hugely from what we unconsciously believe. You may want a healthy lifestyle with your family, where you have time for relaxation and exercise and to prepare and eat healthy food, but if you have a deep-rooted belief that you are not good enough, you may see a pattern of behaviour where you are constantly trying to prove yourself, to the detriment of your goals. For example, you might push hard with your career, working long hours, seeking the next promotion and pay rise, or, you could end up doing all the chores at home and taking on responsibility for everything in family life. Before long, this behaviour can lead to burn out - the exact opposite of what you actually want in life. You are not spending time with your family, you are not taking care of yourself and you are not happy and fulfilled because you are not leading the life you want. Instead, you are leading a life that is in alignment with your belief that you are not good enough.

YOUR FITNESS MINDSET

To create a shift in your subconscious, you must begin by exercising your mind. You do this by becoming aware of your thoughts, words and emotions, rather than focusing on your actions. By gaining awareness of how you operate, you can begin to make changes. Positive, lasting change starts with rewiring your brain. Your language is a clue to your thoughts and what is passing through your mind at any given time. Start paying attention to what you say to yourself. For example, if you are saying: *"I don't have time to exercise"*, ask yourself the following questions:

"What, never?"

"Is this really true all the time?"

"What would happen if you did have time?"

"What needs to happen for you to have the time?"
Or, is the deeper belief here something along the lines of *"One day I'll have time."* The key is to observe the thoughts you are experiencing without judgement. When you want to exercise, but hesitate or put it off, what image is coming up for you about this experience? Notice the feelings this image brings up for you. There is a point at which your brain will produce a cue that says, *"I'm not going to do that now"*. Any picture or feelings that come up at this stage are an insight into what's underneath your procrastination. Often these pictures are not

what you would expect. You are asking your subconscious mind to help you here. It could bring up an image from your childhood, or a recent traumatic event, or simply an experience that was unpleasant. Try to slow down your mental movie of this experience to see what is happening. Being curious about your thoughts is key. Detach yourself from your thoughts and become an observer. You can't control your thoughts, so let them pass, but you can treat your feelings as options, instead of things you have to endure. You can change your emotional response and this is what changes your results. This creates new neural pathways, allowing your brain to choose a better option in future.

CHANGING YOUR NARRATIVE

Expecting your beliefs to disappear overnight isn't reasonable, or practical. Instead, focusing on loosening things up a little gives you more choices. If you have a belief that is proving to be an obstacle to you moving forward with your health and fitness, you can choose to be curious at this stage and learn more about your beliefs and where they have come from. Presumably, you are reading this book because you want to be moving your body more for your health and to look and feel better, so even if you believe exercise is hard (or maybe impossible) for you right now, you know that it is still something you want to achieve, otherwise you wouldn't be complaining about not doing it. When you have discovered what these deep beliefs are, you can start to work on reframing them by simply finding a more positive way of viewing something and shifting your perspective. If one of your beliefs is "*I don't like exercise"*, what thoughts or language can you use instead? How can you reframe your beliefs?

EXAMPLES OF POSITIVE BELIEFS

- My body needs to move to help me feel good.
- My body deserves to be healthy and strong.
- I will nurture my body because it allows me to do so much in life.
- I feel energised after exercise.
- Exercise improves my mood and makes me more pleasant to be around.
- I love feeling my muscles getting stronger and stronger.

You can explore what you would rather believe. This helps you to develop positive habits that will support the achievement of your goals, so good behaviour becomes second nature. Success is now not just achievable, but easy.

YOUR BODY IS YOUR BEST FRIEND

Try this out.

"My body is my best friend." Think about a friend that you very rarely see from one month (or year) to the next. You love this friend dearly and when you see each other, nothing has really changed, and it's like you picked up from where you left off. But if you were to completely cut ties with this friend and never have any contact, the friendship would probably die over time. It would become awkward. You need to nurture this friendship – by text message, or phone call, or going for a drink or dinner together, or perhaps a weekend away. Each of these steps deepens your connection with your friend. If you don't have time for a weekend away, maybe dinner is the best

option right now. But if life is very hectic, a text message is still going to let that person know you care and that they are in your thoughts. If we return to seeing your body as your friend, you need to nurture this relationship in the same way. If you don't have time for an hour-long workout (the equivalent to dinner with your friend), try completing a 15-minute workout instead (the phone call). If that is a stretch on some days, do a one-minute plank, or some star jumps, or plies, or perhaps some rises up and down onto the balls of your feet while you brush your teeth (the text message). This way, you are maintaining a connection with your body. You are nurturing it so each time you go to exercise, it becomes less awkward and instead, enjoyable.

YOUR TENDENCY AND YOUR BELIEFS

Understanding your deep-rooted beliefs helps you to become aware of why you act and why you don't act, as does an understanding of your Tendency. Gaining more awareness around your beliefs and your Tendency can illuminate the hidden aspects of your nature and what has been holding you back in the past. By better understanding your reasons for doing things according to your Tendency, you can start to see how some of your beliefs may have formed in the first place. This could be because a parent or teacher didn't fully understand you as a child and inappropriately labelled you lazy, stubborn, delicate, or clumsy. Or because you didn't have an understanding of what makes you tick either and you reached the same conclusion based on life experiences that made you feel different to others. When it comes to exercise, this new understanding of both your limiting beliefs and your Tendency can allow you to put self-loathing and guilt to one side and enable you to start devising new ways to trick yourself into exercising.

TENDENCY	BELIEF	TAKEAWAY
Upholder	• Your previous failed attempts at exercise are because you didn't plan and schedule it into your diary and your limiting beliefs kept you safe and in your comfort zone. • Articulate your goals clearly and trust in your ability to achieve them.	Stick to the plan and maintain a structure.
Questioner	• Your previous failed attempts at exercise are because the personal health benefits were not top of mind and old beliefs were getting in the way. • You love customisation, so experiment with different forms of movement until you find what works for you. • Spot when you are making excuses not to exercise!	Educate yourself on, and believe there are personal health benefits to exercise and be prepared to try something new.
Obliger	• You deserve to put yourself before others without guilt. • Your previous attempts at exercise failed because you didn't have the right accountability, not because you are in some way flawed.	Believe you are worth it.
Rebel	• Focus on why exercise has personal value to you today, not on what you may have believed in the past. • Think about what you want to gain from exercise and why you want this benefit. • See exercise as a way to express who you are and ditch any other limiting beliefs that may be holding you back.	Be true to yourself and believe exercise is your choice.

Once you are aware of your beliefs and how they have been holding you back, you can begin to reframe the way you view exercise and start to use different language to help rewire your brain for success. At the same time, you will be discovering the right strategies for you to use for consistent exercise, according to your Tendency.

CHAPTER SUMMARY

- Our beliefs about exercise affect our ability to achieve our fitness goals. They can create unhelpful habits that are difficult to break.
- They may come from unpleasant past experiences that your brain - particularly your subconscious - tried to protect you from repeating.
- You can change unhelpful beliefs once you have properly identified them.
- Once you've identified who you are and the exercise identity you want to reinforce, you can choose how to behave to create new habits that will support and reinforce that exercise identity.
- This requires effort, patience and courage - it is easier to go down the well-trodden path on autopilot.
- Becoming more self-aware will allow you to stop being controlled by limiting thoughts and emotions.
- Listen to your inner voice to begin changing your emotional responses, and thereby your actions and results, ultimately leading to new, positive habits.

- Once you understand your beliefs and how they have been holding you back, as well as your Tendency, you can start discussing new ways to trick yourself into exercising and start using different language to help rewire your brain.

NEXT STEPS:

To bring more awareness to your beliefs around exercise, take your time to answer the following questions in your notebook:

1. What are your beliefs as you think about your goal of exercising regularly?
2. What are the beliefs that help you?
3. What are the beliefs that hinder you?
4. When you think about these beliefs, put them into the following statements:

"I can because…"

"I can't because…"

Write all of them until there are no more reasons why you can't.

For these "I can't because" statements, allocate an emotional charge (on a scale of 1-10, 10 being high and 1 being low). Starting with the most emotionally charged statement:

1. Write down all the reasons that this limiting belief is untrue. Let this evidence really sink in until you know that this belief is not true and is not based on reality.
2. Next, replace this limiting belief with one of your "I can..." statements. Use the evidence from above to bolster this belief. Let go of the limiting belief, see it for what it is, and start believing this new positive belief in both your heart and mind.

You can add your "I can because" statements to a vision Board, or use them as affirmations, or journal prompts to remind yourself of your new beliefs every day.

5

FINDING HARMONY WITH YOUR VALUES

Years ago, my values were certainly not top of mind. It wasn't until I had a near death experience, in New York on my 30th birthday, that I took the time to reassess my life. During my ten years as a lawyer in London, I had started to let the things I loved fall away. I was chained to my desk for long hours every day, I didn't have time to think about my wellbeing and for a period of time, I stopped dancing altogether.

The day I turned 30 was the day that changed the course of my life completely. I was on holiday in New York with my best friend, walking home from dinner around 6.30pm. We were metres away from our hotel lobby when a hooded man approached us and put a gun to our heads, demanding we give him all our cash. I had none. My friend had $1.50 and a Macy's card. He didn't believe me. He became more and more agitated and got closer until the gun was practically touching my forehead. Then, he demanded we turn our backs to him. Terrified, we did as we were told. Thankfully, it wasn't the end we feared. He disappeared and we were soon safe. But this brief encounter would alter my life's path entirely. I realised that working as a lawyer meant I was not living life according to my values.

I needed to try and find a better way of living my life for the sake of my mental health and wellbeing. I knew exercise was an important part of that. This set me on a path to reconnect with my passion and train to become a dance teacher, and ultimately, to set up Breaking Ballet. Now I'm living in alignment with my values.

WHY ARE MY VALUES IMPORTANT FOR EXERCISE?

Values are basic and fundamental beliefs, or preferences, that are unique to you, that guide, or motivate your attitudes, or actions. They are your code for life, your principles, the things you hold most dear, your standards of behaviour (what you consider to be right or wrong), and they help you to figure out what is important to you.

As a child, your parents and teachers pass values on to you and you continue to live your life based on what they've taught you is important, whether that be kindness, patience, friendship, etc. But as an adult, you can decide what is of most value to you as an individual. Some of the values from childhood may stay the same, but you may find that others have become increasingly important as you have grown and changed. Tolerance, gratitude, mental and physical health, and family, for example, may be of huge significance to you now. Or, you may find that some values have become less important because they don't really resonate with you personally anymore. But what you value most highly will be clearly apparent in your behaviour and daily routine.

What is most important to you in your life right now?

This is hugely important to the lifestyle changes that you are considering making when committing to a fitness journey. Having a clear idea of what is important to you enables you to prioritise and make daily choices that are in alignment with those things. We must make choices that reflect our values and temperament.

EXAMPLES OF VALUES YOU MAY CURRENTLY HAVE MIGHT BE:

- Being fit enough to play with your children, or grandchildren
- To have a successful business / career
- Spending time with your family
- Travelling
- Having fun
- Getting enough sleep
- Being a good role model
- Feeling confident in your relationship
- Maintaining a certain physique / healthy weight

It's important to have a very clear understanding of what's important to you, so you can see how these values could be either beneficial or problematic for your wellbeing.

Clear decision-making

When you come across the need to make a decision, your values can help you make the right one. Let's say you are busy working at your desk, feeling overwhelmed with emails, calls, client deadlines, billing and admin, all under time pressure, and you just can't see the wood for the trees. You decide to take a short break and stretch your legs and head to the office kitchen to make a cup of tea. Someone at work has brought in a box of doughnuts to share with everyone for their birthday. You want a doughnut, but you are not particularly hungry and have been trying not to eat unhealthy snacks between meals. But you are stressed. You tell yourself you deserve the dough-nut. You have been 'good' for days and today you really need it. You persuade yourself to take the doughnut as it would be rude not to when someone has brought them into the office to share.

This is an example of how our emotions can get in the way of good decision-making, but if you stop to ask yourself, *"What would someone who values health do in this situation?"* then you just might be able to come to a more clear-headed, less emotionally-affected decision.

Eliminating excess baggage

Identifying your values will help you rule out the things you really do not want, need, or believe are important. As a busy woman, you will be fire-fighting most of the time. Racing from one task to the next, ticking off all the chores on your to-do list. You might be ferrying children around to all their activities, looking after elderly parents, providing a shoulder to cry on for a friend whose relationship has broken down, or supporting a family member through a health crisis. All while trying to hold down your own job and running a house. You are on automatic pilot again.

In order to achieve some time and space for your own wellbeing, you will need to let go of some of the tasks in your week to make space for you. We will talk more about the impact of not doing so, as well as how to create new habits and let go of old ones, in later chapters, but tuning into your values will help you to decide now on the areas that are *not* important to you and can be let go.

Do you really need to do all the things you are doing? Can someone else do them? Or can you let go of some of them completely? If you find yourself constantly racing around and never getting to the end of your to-do list, you need to let go!

Building confidence in who you are

Identifying your values increases your level of confidence because it brings about a sense of stability and safety to your life. When you truly know what you want and hold sacred it doesn't matter what other people want. When you know what is important to you, it doesn't matter what is important to other people. This will naturally bring a sense of confidence to your life.

Knowing your values means you can develop confidence to have strong opinions about important subjects. You don't want to just believe what your parents believed. It is your choice now and if necessary, you can stand out from the crowd. You don't have to believe what your friends or family believe. By figuring out what you *truly* believe, you can share your honest self with others. This, in turn, helps you to set healthy boundaries, in order to protect the time you will be carving out for you. Yes, it may upset people, but the sooner you manage their expectations, the better.

Role modelling

There are always two paths we can take in life. One is the path we "should" take (based on other people's expectations) and the second is the path we "want" to take. "Want" in the sense of matching our values - not just "in the moment" hedonistic desires. We must always take the path we want to take, that is in alignment with our values and how we want to show up in this world. And never is that more true than now for health and fitness. It is not a selfish path. It is a smart one. Don't choose to exercise because you think you "should" do so, or restrict your diet because someone told you that you "should" lose a few pounds. Changing the narrative around health and fitness is the only way you will be consistent in your efforts.

In Glennon Doyle's book, Untamed, she describes a conversation with her daughter, Tish.

Tish: *Chase wants me to join the same club he joined in middle school. I don't want to.*

GD: *So don't.*

Tish: *But I don't want to disappoint him.*

GD: *Listen. Every time you're given a choice between disappointing someone else and disappointing yourself, your duty is to disappoint that someone else. Your job, throughout your entire life, is to disappoint as many people as it takes to avoid disappointing yourself.*

Tish: *Even you?*

GD: *Especially me.*

This is a wonderful example of instilling values in children to put themselves first instead of people pleasing. And you can apply the same principle to yourself.

So many women I know have very little time to exercise, or do any self-care, because they are running around after everyone else. I'm not saying we shouldn't take time to help others - I really do believe that we are on this planet to serve others - but not at the expense of our own wellbeing.

Do you remember how people talked about exercise when you were growing up? Did you hear a parent, sibling, friend say "I *have* to go and workout now", or was it "uncool" at school to take part in sport?

If we can instill in the next generation a value of health, they are never going to feel like exercise is something they *should* be doing. It will become something they "can" do because they are choosing to live a long life, full of energy and vitality. It's part of who they are and what they do. And, of course, the best way of instilling this value is by role modelling it.

If you have children, talk to them about how important exercise is to you. Carve out time in your schedule for exercise and tell them that's what you're doing. Invite them to join you if you want to, or tell them to leave you alone for half an hour if you don't. Whatever works for you. And whatever you want them to consider "normal" when they reach adulthood.

I know that if I tell my children they need to get out and move their bodies, and list the multiple reasons why they "should" be exercising, they are going to roll their eyes at me, turn the other way and open up their iPad. But if I show them how I'm honouring my health values by working out, walking in nature, eating healthy foods, getting good quality sleep, and resting when I need to, they are far more likely to take on board these associated behaviours later in life.

WHAT IF I DON'T KNOW WHAT MY VALUES ARE?

You may never have considered what your values are, or how they relate to, or can help motivate you to exercise (or achieve any other life goals), but they are there anyway and will have been helping to determine your behaviour so far in life. You will just have been less aware of it.

You may find that you sometimes struggle to achieve your health and fitness goals because it has always been purely down to chance whether or not the goals, or the steps you have taken to achieve those goals, are aligned to your core values. We want to be able to remove this game of chance, create some certainty, and move forward with intention and purpose. Otherwise, we are at risk of living our lives, or continuing to live our lives, in a way that is incongruent with our core values. This incongruence creates inner turmoil.

One of my clients, Emma, a lawyer in her early 40s with two children, wanted a better work/life balance. She was working long hours, but progressing in her career, something that had always been important to her. However, she was exhausted and discontent. She felt guilty about the time she spent working rather than being with her children... but if she spent time with her children she got behind on her work, which created stress. When we looked at her values, family was at the top. Next was health. Career didn't even feature in her list of eight values. This is why she was feeling so discontent with her life. There were some serious decisions that needed to be made and she entered into discussions with her family to see how they could manage this situation.

Sometimes, just looking at things from a different perspective can help you to work through your situation and find a solution. Even if that just means creating stronger boundaries, being more present doing the activities you value. It doesn't mean an entire overhaul of your life. It's the small changes that will make the biggest difference. Emma's goal of a better work / life balance was in alignment with her values and once she discovered this, she was motivated to make the necessary changes.

We need to know *why* we are choosing particular goals and ensure these goals are in alignment with our values. We can use our values to determine our goals, or, once we have set our goals, we can work to ensure the actions we are taking to achieve those goals are in accordance with our values. This is a really important step in making exercise *necessary* (as discussed in Chapter 3.)

HOW YOUR VALUES AFFECT YOUR TENDENCY

The different Tendencies value different things and this is where it gets interesting. Knowing which Tendency you are will help you to learn more about your values and subsequently, the sorts of behaviours you can adopt to reach your goals.

TENDENCY	VALUES	TAKEAWAY
Upholder	• You value self-command. You don't allow your emotions to drive your choices and you remain in control. • For exercise, implement a regular and predictable workout plan and follow through with it. • You can stay consistent with your exercise to achieve your goal.	Implement your exercise plan undeterred.
Questioner	• You value reason, research and information. • Base your decisions to exercise on information and reason. • Understand why you are exercising. • You need a personal reason to exercise.	Gather all the information you need to build your exercise routine.
Obliger	• You place high value on meeting commitments to others. • Ensure your exercise involves a commitment you have made to someone else, such as a fitness buddy or personal trainer. • Accountability is key for you.	Make a commitment to someone else in relation to your exercise.
Rebel	• You place high value on freedom, choice, identity and self-expression. • Make exercise your choice. • You value pleasure, so choose a form of exercise you enjoy, or see exercise as something that will make you feel good and improve your sex life.	You are free to choose the exercise regime you want to do.

HOW TO REFRAME YOUR HABITS AROUND YOUR VALUES

Whatever your values are in relation to your health and fitness, whether that is physical, mental, or emotional wellbeing, or setting a healthy example for your children, the important question is, do your actions back that up? What are you doing on a daily basis that provides evidence for these values? Perhaps not as much as you think! We are living, breathing manifestations of our values and the way we behave, interact and respond is completely based around the values we hold.

As you can see from my experience on my 30th birthday in New York, my values hadn't necessarily changed over time, but I was able to reframe my thoughts and behaviours around the values that were now so much clearer to me.

If health is one of your top values, but you are not currently taking consistent action towards optimising your health, you can now start to reframe your habits in accordance with those values. But you don't have to change your habits completely. All you need to do if you want to get fitter and healthier is find a way to balance the changes you feel you could make with your values.

For example, if relaxation is an important value for you, and you currently drink wine to help you relax when things are stressful at work, giving up wine may not work unless you find an alternative way to unwind and therefore maintain your value of relaxation.

Equally, if career success to ensure you can look after your family is your most important value, it can be hard to find time to fit exercise and healthy eating into your daily routine. Recognising that being fitter and healthier can help you achieve career success through increased energy, concentration, and motivation is an important step, as is making changes that still allow you to work as hard as you feel is needed.

Consider your five most important values. Might they in any way negatively impact your health, fitness, and wellbeing? Do they positively impact your health, fitness, and wellbeing at all? How might being fitter and healthier help you to live more in line with your values?

Being able to link any lifestyle changes back to your personal values can be a fantastic tool to motivate you to stick at them and maybe even make more changes in future.

So, pack away the guilt and get moving to improve your health and to show the next generation what to do when you value your health.

CHAPTER SUMMARY

- Values are your core beliefs - your standards of behaviour that help you decide what is important in your life.
- Whether you're aware of them or not, your values have been determining your actions throughout your life.

- Identifying your core values, especially regarding your health and fitness, will help you prioritise and make choices that align with your values so you can be true to yourself. This will help you be confident that you are living how you want to live.
- Like it or not, if you have kids, you are a role model for them and both consciously and unconsciously, they will be affected by what you say and do - not just to or with them, but with others and for yourself.
- If you don't demonstrate that it's important to put yourself first, especially around your health and fitness, that's what your kids will see. Is that the behaviour you want them to repeat when they grow up?
- Your values can help you set your goals, or identify actions that will achieve your goals, in accordance with your values.
- Coupled with knowledge of your Tendency, you can better understand your values and identify behaviours that will achieve your goals.

NEXT STEPS

This simple exercise will help you to identify your core values in relation to your health and fitness. Think about your reason for reading this book and your desire for health and fitness:

Step 1: Grab a piece of paper and a pen and just write, just keep writing. What is important to you about achieving greater health and fitness? Then ask yourself why - why is that important? And keep writing. Every time you write something down, think "what else?". Why else is this important? And keep going until you completely run out of ideas.

Step 2: The next thing I would like you to do is choose somewhere between eight and 10 of the values you have identified. From everything that you've just written down, you might start to notice some common themes. If you've got a desire to lose weight, one of the values might be confidence. *"I want to feel confident. That's really important to me."*

Step 3: Looking at your list, are there any values that mean the same thing? Can you remove any duplicate values, or combine them?

Step 4: Choose which value you see as the most important. Now order the list in order of importance.

Step 5: Check that you have the list in the correct order by taking the top value and asking yourself, *"If I could have this value (first value) but couldn't have the second value on my list, would that be okay?"* If it's not ok, you need to swap those values around. For example, if my value one is confidence and my value two is health, I'm asking myself, if I can have confidence but not health, is that ok? The answer is "no". So I will move "health" to the top of the list and "confidence" will become second on my list.

Step 6: Repeat the above step going down your list (*"If I can have value 1 but not value 3, is that ok?"*) until you determine which value has a priority over the others.

EXAMPLES OF SOME HEALTH AND FITNESS VALUES ARE:		
Calmness	Balance	Energy
Fun	Challenge	Longevity
Strength	Positivity	Eating nutritious food
Joy	Determination	Healthy ageing
Happiness	Wellbeing	Time in nature
Confidence	Coping	Flexibility

6

GOALS - HEADING IN THE RIGHT DIRECTION

In the next two chapters we are going to look at your health and fitness goals and how to create the right habits to achieve them. I won't be telling you what your goals "*should*" be, or what you "*should*" focus on. This will depend on your motivation, beliefs, and values, as just discussed. Your goals are none of my business (or anyone else's for that matter) and you can allow it to be a very private process if you want to (unless you are an Obliger, in which case you may benefit from sharing your goals to get the accountability you need).

Goal setting is important because it provides us with direction and helps us to prioritise behaviours that will help us reach our desired outcome. Goals can give us a purpose and a plan and drive us forward to progress, or in some way improve ourselves. When it comes to fitness, setting goals means we are better able to hold ourselves accountable; they motivate us to move, show us what we are capable of and push us outside our comfort zone.

NO SHAME ALLOWED

I talk a lot about moving your body first and foremost in order to prioritise your health, but if your goal is an aesthetic one (losing a few pounds around your mid-section, developing toned arms, or fitting into your jeans), that's absolutely fine. Please don't feel any shame if you have ever, or are currently, prioritising the numbers on the scale, or the label in your jeans over your health. Frankly, it doesn't matter what's motivating you right now provided it's meaningful to you, which we will talk about shortly. Ultimately, I want you to be moving and hopefully enjoying the process so you continue to move for the rest of your life. This way, you will experience the myriad of health benefits that movement brings, including its side effects - weight loss, a toned body, and youthful appearance.

The problem starts when continued focus on how you look becomes your ONLY reason for moving. In my experience, this can mean that exercise is unsustainable over the long term, because you are likely to stop moving once you have reached your goal (a certain weight, for example), or because you fail to achieve your goal in the timescale you set (perhaps the bar was set too high in the first place), or you don't feel any better about how you are actually living your life.

DEVELOPING A HEALTH STANDARD

Considering what has influenced your choice of goal may help to avoid some of these pitfalls. For example, is your chosen goal influenced by your social environment - the people you spend time with, or the images you are exposed to on social media? What standards are you trying to live up to? Is it a health standard of fitness (reducing your risk of cardiovascular disease, or diabetes, for example), or an athletic standard (like a Cross Fit competition), or is it a body beautiful standard? There are many "looks" that trend at different times, and different cultures have different body standards. For example, in American culture the "ideal" woman's body is the "Barbie" look - skinny and surgically enhanced. But there are some cultures in Nigeria who would consider a larger woman healthier and more beautiful. Women's body standards in Western cultures are typically set by the media.

If you don't like a particular body standard of fitness, you are less likely to participate in exercise if that means complying with that standard. On the other hand, if you are working towards a health standard, this can eliminate any unwillingness because you value your health. If you don't have a health standard at all, this can make you vulnerable to a host of "magic fitness programmes" that are not helpful and sometimes harmful.

THE PROBLEM WITH "NEW YEAR, NEW ME"

Whatever your influences, I'm willing to bet you have, at some point, resolved on 1st January to achieve ALL your wellness goals that year, which meant creating some new habits - moving more, eating less, getting more sleep, creating a work/life balance, having more fun, etc. You may have signed up to the latest fitness trend, started a juice diet, bought some fitness clothing, or equipment, or signed up to an expensive gym membership. Your intentions were good and your desire was strong to maintain this new lifestyle.

Then, by mid-January, the pressure has got to you. Life has scuppered your good intentions and you give up, telling yourself you just don't have it in you. *"This is not the right time. One day it will be easier"*. Then you start to berate yourself for failing to achieve your goals. But there is nothing wrong with you. You just didn't have the right strategy in place. And by the way, there is never a perfect time to start. Something will always come along to challenge you.

This is why goals need to be set up in the right way at the beginning, in accordance with your belief system (motivation, beliefs, values, and identity), so you have a fighting chance of achieving them. The trick is to understand what behaviours are necessary to achieve your goal, and to ensure that these behaviours become habits - actions that we take on a consistent/routine basis towards achieving the outcome we desire.

THE THREE SIMPLE STEPS TO GOAL SETTING

So, let's keep this simple and set up your goals in three simple steps.

1. YOUR DESTINATION GOAL

Your destination goal is your big, end goal. The one thing you would like to achieve above all other goals. There will, of course, be different strategies to get you there, but without deciding on your destination you will either struggle to get started in the first place, or get lost along the way. You may have experienced this first hand when your new year's resolutions fizzled out once again. The key is to understand how we can learn from years of repeatedly performing the same behaviour, expecting a different result.

When creating your destination goal, you will need to have your values at the top of your mind, to ensure your new fitness goal is in alignment with what is truly important to you. This is the big goal that you want to achieve at some time in the future, but for now don't worry about *how* you will get there. We are coming onto that in the next chapter. For the time being, choose a goal that you feel, with the right strategies, you can achieve.

When you have your goal in mind, ask yourself why this goal is important to you. When you are clear on your reasons for setting your particular fitness goal, this will help motivate you to stick with it and keep it in your sights, even when life gets challenging.

EXAMPLES OF DESTINATION GOALS
I want to feel stronger so that I can pick up my child/grandchild without struggling.
I want to lose weight around my mid-section so I feel more body confident.
I want to run 5k in under 30 minutes to help improve my cardiovascular fitness as I age.
I want to strengthen and tone my body to increase my muscle mass, increase my metabolism and protect my bones through perimenopause and beyond.
I want to improve my mobility / flexibility to reduce my aches and pains and avoid injury.

2. PROCESS GOALS

Once you have decided on your destination goal and why this is important to you, the next step is to decide upon the small steps to help you get to your destination goal. These are the daily behaviours you can control. The daily "non-negotiables", as I call them. I ask my clients to choose no more than three non-negotiables to work on at any given time. These can be any behaviours you think will move you towards your destination goal - the mini goals that move you towards your destination goal. These are now your focus on a daily basis. Try to let go of your destination goal for now and instead focus on achieving your mini-goals, or non-negotiables, each day.

Usually, we split these non-negotiables into three categories:

1. *Move* - moving your body.
2. *Nourish* - providing your body with healthy food and keeping it hydrated.
3. *Nurture* - focusing on your mental and emotional wellbeing.

For example, if your destination goal is to tone up your tummy, your process goals might be to:

1. Get up 15 minutes earlier each day to workout;
2. Drink at least 8 glasses of water every day to avoid dehydration and bloating; and
3. Reduce your stress levels by saying *"no"* as many times as you can!

When it comes to improving our fitness, our tradition is to set exercise performance goals - working out three times a week, running 10k at weekends, or lifting a certain weight in the gym. Depending on your Tendency, this commitment to attain a certain performance level in order to achieve your goal can exert a great deal of pressure and lead to overwhelm pretty early on when you realise how unrealistic this goal was at the outset.

Are you being smart?

Another way of looking at goals is the popular SMART acronym for goal setting, which stands for:

*   **Specific:** The goal should be clear and precise, while also serving as a personal motivator.
*   **Measurable:** The goal should be something that can be objectively measured so that you can accurately track progress.
*   **Achievable:** The goal should be realistic enough to obtain, yet challenging enough to push you beyond your regular routine.

- **R**elevant: The goal needs to feel important to you and align with your other fitness-related aspirations.
- **T**ime-bound: This provides a deadline and will help you stay on task and keep the outcome goal a priority.

SMART goals are helpful to break down your goal and ensure that it will work for you, but ironically, it's not always the smartest way to goal-setting. This is because it's missing one vital ingredient in goal setting and habit creation - your 'Why'. So when it comes to setting and implementing your process goals, as well as using the SMART acronym, you also need to have your "why" top of mind. The easiest way to do this is to write down your reason for setting your destination goal, and look at it every time you implement a process goal.

You may have set goals many times before, but if you missed out why you have chosen this particular goal, then it's likely that after a certain period of time, you will not be interested in achieving the goal anymore (cue the new year's resolution trap again). The reason is not lack of motivation, or lack of resources, or the fact you haven't put in the hard work. The reason is you are focused on achieving the outcome instead of focusing on why this is important to you, which doesn't allow you to forge an emotional connection to the goal. It becomes boring and the habits associated with the goal become just another chore on your to-do list.

For example, say Anna wants to lose three stone in weight by the end of the year. At the beginning, she is really motivated and joins a gym on 1st January. She starts working out and eating better. She loses one stone after two months and feels fantastic. Then, in March, she goes on holiday, relaxing on the beach, eating and drinking and having fun. She isn't exercising and arrives home only to realise she has regained a stone and feels terrible, guilty, and defeated. Eventually, she succumbs to her old habits and gives up on her goal. What went wrong?

Minor setbacks can put a big dampener on outcome-focused goals and SMART goals often fail to fuel someone's inner fire. We may be taking all the necessary steps consciously, but our subconscious mind doesn't understand why we are behaving in a certain way. If we can focus on intrinsic motivation, it is much more likely to lead to long-term behaviour change. Obligers and Rebels bear with me.

Your "base acceptable bottom"

If you have felt overwhelmed by goal-setting in the past, it's time to take a different approach. Rather than setting performance goals, which can cause a lot of pressure, you could set a base acceptable bottom. This is your excuse level. It is a level of performance below which you refuse to fall and will not make excuses - even to yourself. For many of us, it is less stressful to avoid failure than to strive to break records. This allows you to be gentle with yourself and grow towards your goal. Slow and steady wins the race! So, rather than trying to set a press-up record every time you workout, set an excuse level of at least half of your personal best. Do that once every week, whether you think you're prepared or not.

The key is to focus on what you can control and take bite-sized steps that feel achievable. These process goals will be your new habits that we will explore further in the next chapter.

3. IMPLEMENTATION

Planning is a really important process and vital to your success. If you don't plan properly, this may well be what has hampered your progress in the past. But planning will amount to nothing unless you take action.

Allow exercise to encroach into your life

We know from discussing your beliefs earlier in this book that lack of time is just a story you are telling yourself to avoid exercising. In most cases (and there are exceptions), it is simply a question of priorities. Or, perhaps the real problem is not time alone, but the inability to sustain the time required for fitness even if you are having fun (which, let's face it, is not always the case!).

Many of us can spend an hour exercising three days a week for a short while. But sustaining it for five years is a problem. An obvious solution is to shorten the time we are working out. All the ballet-inspired workouts I deliver to clients are 10-15 minutes long. But I'm not sure that shortening the time alone is as effective at sustaining the lifestyle as increasing the frequency to 5-7 days per week, alongside reducing your workout time.

This frequency means that exercise encroaches into your life. Don't you think it would be psychologically easier to find five days a week to do 15 minutes of exercise than to find one hour three days per week? With the latter, you have four days to find an excuse to miss one of your three exercise days. If you are sitting on the fence every day, deciding whether today will be one of the three days you exercise, this leads to decision fatigue and procrastination. If you reduce your time working out, and increase your frequency, this will raise your fitness level.

I can already hear you ask *"But doesn't my body need a break from working out to avoid injury?"*. Well, if your workouts damage your body by working out 5-7 days a week, perhaps you need to find another workout, or modify the ones you have so you are working different body parts on different days to avoid injury through fatigue. Remember, we are always paying attention and listening to what our body needs and adapting as we go.

Schedule it in your diary

Not long ago, a lady sent me a message explaining that she had no time to exercise. She got up at 4am to drive two hours to work, worked for ten hours straight and then drove the two hours home again. THIS is someone who is struggling for time to workout. Unless you are doing the same, there are ways you can fit exercise into your busy schedule. We are all busy women, but this can't be an excuse for not prioritising our health and fitness.

Exercising daily is the best way to keep the habit sustainable for me; you have to choose what works for you. Remember, we are all different. These are just suggestions and perhaps a different way of looking at things. Whatever you decide, I believe that it's important for you to schedule exercise into your diary, just like you would any other appointment. I know, I know. Life doesn't always go to plan. But just think how much more likely you are to complete your workout if you have it planned in, than if you are just winging it and hoping it will happen.

To help you with this, use a table similar to the one below. First, highlight the blocks where you are busy. You could use different colours for different activities, like household chores, meetings, taxiing the kids to classes, work, cooking, or socialising. This is to identify where in your week you have free time to put your daily goals into practice. Discover what time of day you have identified as free. Or, if you are struggling to identify any time, rearrange some of the blocks to make time. Do you really need to be doing three rounds of laundry a week, or spending 45 minutes a day tidying the house? You only need 15 minutes for a workout. Carve out this time for YOU and put boundaries around it.

	Monday	Tuesday	Wednesday	Thursday	Friday	Saturday	Sunday
5.00							
6.00							
7.00							
8.00							
9.00							
10.00							
11.00							
12.00							
13.00							
14.00							
15.00							
16.00							
17.00							
18.00							
19.00							
20.00							
21.00							
22.00							
23.00							

If you can press pause and take a moment to look at your schedule, you can find a way to be consistent with your fitness. By *making* time, rather than trying to *find* it, you will feel more empowered. Admittedly, sometimes we have to be creative with when and what we are doing, but there has to be time somewhere in our day when we can move. First thing in the morning is a wonderful time to schedule your exercise as a recurring appointment. This time of the day is usually protected from any distractions, or interruptions. As long as you are getting to bed at a decent hour and sleeping between 7-8 hours, set your alarm to get up early and workout. The benefits last all day long.

CHAPTER SUMMARY

- Goal setting is important because it gives us direction and helps us prioritise behaviours to achieve the goal.
- But your goals need to be carefully set up to match what you really want/need so that they are realistic and achievable in all the circumstances. Otherwise, you are setting yourself up for failure.
- Start by setting your ultimate destination goal. Once you've identified that, ask yourself <u>why</u> that's the end goal. There will be an immediate, superficial "why" you want to achieve that goal, but dig deeper and deeper until you identify the true base reason behind the goal. Anchoring your goal to this base "why" will help you retain focus on what really matters and improve your chances of success because you will have an emotional connection to achieving your goal.
- Next, set the goals or targets that you will meet on the way to achieve your destination goal. Make them SMART goals - the "A" (achievable) is really important here. It may help to have a main SMART goal, but also

a base acceptable bottom - the level of performance below which you refuse to fall.

- These are the daily behaviours you can control. By making them simple and achievable, you can help turn them into habits, so that they become second-nature rather than conscious chores.
- The simplest approach is to split them into three categories - move, nourish, nurture - developing them over time as you get fitter and stronger.
- Ultimately, you must implement your plan. Little but often is likely to be the most effective approach - aim for 15 minutes a day, five days or more a week, at the same time each day. That will help you form habits more easily.
- Put it in your diary - if it's in your smartphone you can even set up an alarm to remind you to get going.

NEXT STEPS

You'll set your process goals (the stepping stones to achieving the destination goal) in the next chapter, which looks at creating good habits. At this stage, you will focus on setting your destination goal.

YOUR DESTINATION GOAL

1. Make a list of your fitness goals. Write down all that you have ever wanted to achieve.

2. Score each goal on a scale of 1-10, 10 being the goal that has the highest emotional charge for you. The one goal you would really like to achieve.

3. Is your chosen goal something that feels achievable if you had the right strategies? Look at the SMART goals again. Also, look at your Greatest Hits - do you have evidence of being able to achieve what you set your mind to? (See Chapter 3)

4. Next, think about the reason you want to achieve this goal. What is your "why"? Look at your personal motivators. (See Chapter 3)

5. What positive beliefs can you use to support you in achieving this goal? (See Chapter 4)

Along with the suggestions above, here are some questions that may also help you when you start to look at goal setting:

1. What specifically do you want? State this desire in the positive.

2. What is your reason for choosing this goal? What is important to you about achieving greater health and fitness (i.e., your values)?

3. Where are you now? What is your present situation?

4. When you have achieved this goal what will you see, hear, feel and say to yourself?

5. What will this outcome get for you, or enable you to do?

6. How will you know when you have achieved your goal?

7. Is this goal only for you?

8. Where, when, and with whom do you want it?

9. What do you have now and what do you need to achieve your outcome?

10. Have you ever had or done this before? Or do you know anyone who has? (Can you act as if you have it?)

11. For what purpose do you want this? What will you gain or lose if you have it?

SMALL CHANGES MAKE THE BIGGEST DIFFERENCES

I t is very common when it comes to achieving your health and fitness goals to want to do a complete overhaul, change everything at once and try to become a "whole new person". But this approach is risky and inevitably leads to us falling from a great height if we don't manage to live up to our own expectations. In the short term, it's far more important for you to show yourself how you can stick to a plan, rather than make huge changes overnight.

In the last chapter, we looked at what process goals are - the evolving stepping stones to achieving the destination goal. Now let's look at how to create those process goals and how to make them easier to achieve by turning them into habits you perform automatically.

WHAT IS A HABIT?

A habit is a behaviour that is repeated regularly and that you often decide to do subconsciously. The life you are living today is largely the sum of your habits to this point. How fit you are today is a result of your exercise habits to date.

Decisions are demanding for your brain. If you've ever felt mentally exhausted after a day full of meetings, then you know what I mean. This causes a problem when it comes to your fitness. There are many decisions involved to begin with, like, *"What exercises shall I do today? When shall I do them? How long shall I do them for? What shall I wear? Where shall I do them? Do I have enough time?"*.

Putting yourself through this mental overload uses up the same pool of resources that you need to show the willpower and self-control to do things like go to the gym. In other words, making hard decisions at work, deciding whether or not to go to the gym, and saying no to that piece of cake, all compete for the same pool of mental resources. The question is, how do we solve this little problem? The answer is: by creating a habit.

When something is repeated often enough, the decision to perform that task moves to a part of your brain called the basal ganglia. Once there, the decision is processed in the background and no longer requires a costly, conscious decision. This is what's known as a "habit".

Discipline is the skill that allows us to create a habit - to stop using up mental energy in making conscious decisions to exercise. You do this by repeating a task over and over again—going to the gym at the same time every day, deciding to do your online workout early every morning, preparing tomorrow's meals at the end of every day, etc. Habits require willpower at the start, but it is a smart and useful utilisation of willpower. Discipline allows us to use willpower as the "battery" that starts the car, as opposed to the energy source that keeps it going. But what happens when you allow your habits to direct you towards a behaviour that you don't want, or is not helpful to you?

How many times have you been asked to do something for someone and even though you really don't have time, you have agreed to help, which has left you feeling resentful, tired, stressed, and overwhelmed? You don't feel comfortable saying no!

Or, you may be able to recall a situation where someone triggers a response in you. Perhaps your mother innocently comments on the way you prepare your child's food, or on what you are wearing, and within seconds, you feel agitated or hurt. Afterwards, you may realise that this reaction changes nothing about the situation and that you can instead choose to remain happy and relaxed. But in the moment, it is very challenging to get this perspective and control your old familiar pattern.

Remember Pavlov's dogs? In the 1890s, the young Russian scientist strapped a few dogs to a table, rang a bell and then fed dogs a good meal. Over time, after repeatedly exposing the dogs to the same stimulus, he simply rang the bell and the dogs automatically salivated in anticipation. This is called a conditioned response and it's an automatic process. This is why it is so hard to change. Your body responds automatically with little conscious effort.

When you are on autopilot, your mind doesn't get to choose anymore. You are operating solely out of habit because your brain is trying to protect you. It is trying to avoid possible negative, or lower vibrating emotions (e.g., frustration, anxiety, anger, sadness). When you feel stuck in the same old patterns, it is because your brain is in survival mode. Your brain believes your old habits are central to your survival and it will create strong urges for you to act a certain way in order to ensure you maintain your current habits. Your subconscious tries to block any unpleasant past experiences by altering your behaviour, which can result in negative outcomes like procrastination, conformism, overthinking, anxiety, or imposter syndrome.

Imagine a well-trodden pathway through a forest. This is the easiest path to follow and the one that many people go down over and over again. So you follow it too. If you wanted to create a new path in a different direction, it would require effort, patience, and courage. You are not sure where this new path goes. It is much easier to go down a path that has already been made. This is you on autopilot.

This autopilot can also contribute to limiting beliefs that can run your life and alter what you perceive. Your capacity for self-awareness and reflection enables you to investigate yourself. It enables you to plan how you will change your behaviour so that you are able to achieve your goals. Your attention is where you place your energy.[1]

JUST 1% IMPROVEMENT

With regard to creating habits to help improve our health and fitness, it's tempting to believe that massive success (losing a lot of weight, running a marathon, increasing our tone or flexibility) requires massive action. We put pressure on ourselves to make some huge improvement that will have everyone talking. We forget that whilst we are not our behaviours (we have the power to change), our current circumstances are a direct result of all the tiny behaviours we have adopted over the years until now. The things that we tell ourselves won't make a difference (one biscuit with our cup of tea, just one glass of wine when the kids have gone to bed, skimping on sleep, or snacking late at night) all add up and we can see and feel the effects of those habits, some of which seem to creep up on us unexpectedly.

But the same is true when we come to implementing healthy habits to drive us towards our goal. You don't see change overnight. Sometimes you don't notice any change at all! But it is more meaningful in the long run. The difference a tiny improvement can make over time is staggering. If you can get 1% better each day for one year, you'll end up thirty-seven times better by the time you're finished.[2] What starts as a small win accumulates into something much, much more. Small habits have a huge return on our lives.

The effects of our habits don't seem to have a huge effect on any given day and yet the impact they make over months, or years, is enormous. It's only when you look back two, five, or 10 years later that the value of good habits becomes apparent. But this is why creating healthy habits can feel difficult. We are so used to instant gratification that when we don't experience this, and achieve our goals within the timescale we have set, it can lead us to give up altogether.

This is the beginning of you making choices that are just 1% better than the choices you made yesterday, and it is these choices that will determine the difference between who you are today and who you could become. Success is the product of daily habits, not once in a lifetime transformations.

THE SCIENCE

I'll keep this explanation short, but it is important to understand how habits work and how to improve them. Your brain will run through a four step pattern every time you build a habit - cue, craving, response, and reward. If your behaviour has all four of these steps, you have created a habit.

1. **Cue, or trigger**. This triggers your brain to initiate the behaviour. This bit of information predicts a reward (a primary reward like food, water, or sex, or a secondary reward like money, fame, praise, approval, friendship, or some form of personal satisfaction). This naturally leads to a craving for the reward.

2. **Craving**. This is the motivational force behind every habit. What you crave is not the habit itself, but the change in state that it brings.

3. **Response**. This is the behaviour you perform, which can be a thought or an action. Depending on how much effort is required, or how capable you feel, will dictate whether you follow through with the behaviour.

4. **Reward**. The response delivers a reward which marks the end of the goal. The reward satisfies the craving and tells us which actions are worth remembering.

If any part of this four step pattern is insufficient, our behaviour won't become a habit. For example, if there is no cue we will never start. If there is no craving we have no motivation. If the behaviour is difficult, we won't be able to do it and if the reward doesn't satisfy us, we won't do it again. Without all four steps, a behaviour will not be repeated and will therefore not become a habit.

WORKED EXAMPLE OF 4-STEP HABIT CREATION FOR EXERCISING IN THE MORNING

1. Cue - you wake up.
2. Craving - you want to exercise because it will help you lose weight and improve your cardiovascular fitness and stamina (your goal is to run a 5k). This improved fitness and weight loss will make you feel accomplished, happier, stronger and more energised. You also want to be a good role model to your children and show them that it's important to prioritise your health and wellbeing (your "why").
3. Response - you complete the workout.
4. Reward - you satisfy your craving to feel accomplished, happier, stronger, and more energised. Working out becomes associated with waking up.

If you are wondering why you are not achieving your goal, the answer lies somewhere in these four steps. These steps influence nearly everything we do each day. But the key is in harnessing these four steps into a practical framework that you can use to create good habits.

Each time you complete a behaviour using this framework, a new neural pathway is created in your brain. Every time you repeat the behaviour, the neural pathway is strengthened and becomes easier to access. This is why your first few workouts feel harder, but after a few months, you're in a routine and finding it much easier. You have rewired your brain to create a positive habit of exercise.

THE FOUR SIMPLE STEPS TO HABIT CREATION

Using the four steps, we can now create a practical framework to design new habits and break old ones. We are going to look at your process goals and how you can turn them into habits. In his book, "Atomic Habits", James Clear calls this the Four Laws of Behaviour Change. To create good habits we need to take a look at the above pattern and:

- Make the cue (to exercise) obvious;
- Make the craving attractive;
- Make the response (behaviour) easy; and
- Make the reward satisfying.

1. MAKING THE CUE OBVIOUS

When it comes to creating a habit of exercise, the two most common cues are time and location. If you are *implementing* your goals (step 3 of the goal setting process in Chapter 6), you will be planning in advance when you are going to exercise (scheduling it into your diary) and where you will do so. These are great cues to get you started, especially if you are setting up your physical environment to support the cue by laying out your exercise clothing or equipment in readiness for your workout. Remember, it's not necessarily about motivation, but about gaining clarity over what you need to do.

Another way to make the cue obvious is to use anchoring, sometimes also called habit stacking. This is simply a strategy where you identify a current habit you already do each day and stack, or anchor, your desired habit to that existing habit. In the case of exercise, this could be *"after getting out of bed in the morning, I put on my workout clothes and complete my 15 minute workout"*. Or, *"after I take off my work shoes, I get changed and go for my run"*. Or, *"when I see a set of stairs I will take them instead of the lift"*.

2. MAKING THE CRAVING ATTRACTIVE

Every behaviour that is highly habit forming - drugs, junk food, video games, social media - creates higher levels of dopamine production (the feel good hormone). Dopamine releases not only when you experience pleasure, but when you anticipate it. It is the anticipation of a reward that gets us to take action. Desire is the engine that drives habits, so you are more likely to find a behaviour attractive if you combine it with doing one of your favourite things.

Again, we can use an anchoring technique - linking an action you want to do with an action you need to do. For example, watching Netflix (want) while riding your exercise bike (need). If you want to read more, but need to exercise more, you can decide to complete your workout after you have chosen your book. After you have completed your workout, you can then read your book.

I'm not necessarily an advocate for distracting your mind with other activities while you are working out and much prefer to connect the mind and body in movement, but to do this, you could play your favourite music while you workout, or add in your preferred stretch session at the end of your workout.

3. MAKING THE BEHAVIOUR EASY

We touched on this in the last chapter. Rather than cranking up your motivation, which requires effort, you can make your habits easy by reducing them to their most basic form. For exercise, this might mean starting out by moving for just two minutes instead of 15 minutes. Or, it could mean doing one press up in the morning for a week, just to get you started on creating a simple ritual for yourself, holding the time and space for movement each day with a view to increasing the time and effort once you are ready.

Optimising your physical environment clearly plays an important part here too. Habits are much easier if they fit into the flow of your life. You are more likely to go to the gym if it's on the way to work. Our natural animal instincts are always to look to take the path of least resistance, so shrinking the habit into a tiny habit, or "gateway habit", can reduce any overwhelm or friction.

Tiny dancer

One of the best ways to make exercise feel easy is to scale back the time and effort you spend doing it. If you are able to maintain a habit of exercising for 2 minutes every morning, you can easily increase this time by 10% each day to get you up to 15 minutes of exercise, or more. If you are struggling to do this, finding a stepping stone, or gateway habit that leads you to the habit of exercise can be helpful. For example, if you want to make a habit of completing a ballet-inspired workout each morning, start by getting up 15 minutes earlier each morning. Set your alarm and when it goes off get out of bed. If you don't do the workout that's fine. Keep the bar low. The objective is to start with a crucial step towards your desired habit of exercising. Getting up early will shift your perspective. Working out suddenly won't seem as hard.

Twyla Tharp is a popular American dancer, director, and choreographer and is considered one of America's most important contemporary dance choreographers. She credits much of her success to simple daily habits.

"I begin each day of my life with a ritual. I wake up at 5.30am, put on my workout clothes, my leg warmers, my sweat shirt and my hat. I walk outside my Manhattan home, hail a taxi and tell the driver to take me to the Pumping Iron gym at 91st street and First Avenue, where I work out for 2 hours. The ritual is not the stretching and weight training I put my body through each morning at the gym; the ritual is the cab. The moment I tell the driver where to go, I have completed the ritual. It's a simple act but doing it the same way each morning habitualises it - makes it repeatable, easy to do. It reduces the chance that I would skip it or do it differently. It is one more item in my arsenal of routines and one less thing to think about".

Now, I'm not suggesting you start getting up at 5.30am and make time to workout for 2 hours a day, but you can see from this example how a simple ritual can be a gateway for the habit you want to maintain.

4. MAKING THE REWARD SATISFYING

We know that forging an emotional connection to your goal is critical for success and celebrating your wins is the best way to create a positive feeling that wires in your new habits, but in our modern society, many of the choices you make now will not benefit you immediately (for example, if you exercise now, you won't be overweight next year). Because of the way we have evolved, we place high value on instant gratification. It's interesting that when it comes to "bad" habits (the ones we want to remove), the immediate outcome feels good (the sugar high eating a chocolate brownie), but the ultimate outcome feels bad (weight gain). If you think of the healthy habits you want to create, the immediate outcome is not always enjoyable but the ultimate outcome feels good. As a rule, the more immediate the pleasure, the more strongly you should question whether it aligns with your long-term goals. It really depends on who you want to choose - the future you, or the present you.

The best way to train yourself to delay gratification is to add a little bit of immediate pleasure to the habits that pay off in the long-run.

Feeling successful

As to rewards, we need to make sure that it is an experience that is directly tied to the behaviour, that makes that behaviour more likely to happen again. Taking yourself off for a massage is a lovely way to reward yourself for working out all week, but this is more of an incentive than a reward. And eating a slice of cake as a reward isn't necessarily in alignment with your goals and the identity you are trying to foster.

Using incentives as rewards can sometimes be dangerous for habit formation because they teach you that you wouldn't do the activity for its own sake. You are extrinsically motivated and you are only exercising to get the reward. But this means you then associate exercising with an imposition, or suffering.

If your reward is hitting a finish line, like losing a certain amount of weight, or completing a marathon, this can also undermine habit creation. Once you stop, you will need to start again. And starting to exercise again is much harder than continuing to do so on a regular basis.

The goal is to exercise forever and have the habit weaved into your lifestyle, so the challenge is to make habits rewarding without sabotaging yourself with rewards. This can be done by finding a reward in the habit itself.

Rewards need to happen at the time you are exercising, or seconds afterwards. It is the dopamine release while you are exercising that helps to rewire your brain. One way is to view your exercise as a "treat".[3] Instead of your workout being something you feel you should do, it becomes your treat - your time for yourself during a day that is filled with other responsibilities. In addition, you can reward yourself immediately after the workout with a celebration. Of course, we will all have different likes and dislikes, so you need to find a celebration that works for you. Your brain will then make the habit of exercise more automatic in the future.

So how will you celebrate? A simple smile, saying a quiet affirmation in your head, high fiving your partner, doing a dance, taking a deep breath, putting on your favourite upbeat soundtrack, imagining your future self giving you a pat on the back, or doing a fist pump are all options that can be done immediately after your workout.

I know they don't seem like huge celebrations, but as long as it makes you feel good, creates a feeling of success and feels authentic to you, it will work. You may find celebrating easy, or you may find it awkward to begin with if you are used to being self-deprecating. Take your time and find what works for you. Eventually, an intrinsic reward like better mood, more energy, or reduced stress, kicks in and you will be less concerned with chasing any secondary rewards. Your identity becomes the reinforcer. Seeing yourself as an "exerciser", "runner" etc. will help reinforce your motivation and habits and support you in achieving your goals. This is discussed further in Chapter 9.

WHICH HABITS TO FOCUS ON

As to which habits you decide to create, it really depends on what your destination goal is and what your associated process goals are. But if you are a woman in your 40s and beyond (who may be perimenopausal, or menopausal), there are some key habits that are foundational to improving your physical, mental, and emotional health.

THE FOUR FOUNDATIONS

The focus of this book is on getting you to move more, so unsurprisingly, one of the foundational habits below is exercise. But there are three other habits that not only contribute to a healthier lifestyle, but also have a direct impact on your motivation to exercise. These are sleep, stress management, and nutrition. Remember my Move, Nourish, and Nurture non-negotiables? This is where they come into play, when you are planning out your process goals.

While this book is focused on the exercise element/foundation, the other elements are really important in achieving exercise, health, and fitness success too. I'm not going to go into detail on those here, but recommend you also include process goals and habits around the other foundations to support your success.

1. SLEEP

If you are not getting enough sleep (more than 7 hours a night), you are likely to be prone to putting on weight.[4] You have two hormones in your body that are responsible for regulating your appetite - Leptin, which tells you when you are full, and Ghrelin, which tells you when you are hungry. When you are not getting enough quality sleep there is a decrease in Leptin (so you are not receiving as many messages telling you that you are full) and an increase in Ghrelin (sending more messages telling you that you are hungry). Not ideal. Research shows that lack of sleep increases cravings for sweets, carbohydrate-rich foods and salty snacks by between 30-40%.[5] So next time you have had a rough night, don't be surprised to find yourself at the back of the fridge, reaching for everything and anything that will help satisfy your cravings.

In addition, if you are sleep deprived you are not going to have the energy reserves to exercise and you will be more prone to injury. So, take a look at your bedtime routine and decide what time you need to go to sleep in order to put yourself in the best possible position of getting those 7-8 hours of sleep. I get up at 6am to workout most mornings, so I'm in bed by 9.30pm, reading before lights out at 10pm. This is, of course, becoming more challenging now my children are older and more often than not, it's me nagging them to go to bed so I can do the same! It doesn't always work (especially if I want a night out), but I'm putting myself in the best possible position to achieve my goal.

2. REDUCE STRESS

We know that increased stress causes raised levels of Cortisol (the stress hormone) in the body. If your cortisol levels are high, this disrupts your quantity and quality of sleep. In addition, high cortisol levels will slow down your metabolism, leaving you more likely to put on weight. This is because the body thinks the rise in cortisol levels means it's in danger and automatically goes into its fight, flight, or freeze response. It holds on to fat to protect you (most notably around your midsection to shield your vital organs). There are many ways you can incorporate small self-care habits into your daily life to help reduce your stress levels:

- Daily steps - such as going for a walk, particularly in natural surroundings, like a park or the countryside
- Calm things down - meditation, breathing exercises
- Nourishing your body with wholesome food
- More sleep
- Limited caffeine and alcohol - disrupts sleep and high in sugar
- Gentle movement practices like yoga or tai chi
- Seeking support from others with your goals
- Journaling
- Setting clear boundaries to protect your time alone

- Spending time with friends

3. EAT WELL

It's almost impossible to look at your fitness goals without addressing your nutrition. What you eat, how much you eat, and when you eat is crucial to support your efforts with exercise, both to ensure you have the energy to exercise, but also to help you if your goals include weight loss and/or toning and strengthening your body.

I'm not a nutritionist and the focus of this book is to get you exercising, but it's important to bring your attention to your eating habits at this stage. What you eat is even more important as you enter your 40s. As you age, you start to lose muscle mass, your metabolism drops and you may gain weight. Your diet can help to mitigate these negative effects of ageing.

Women need protein (meat, fish, eggs, dairy, beans and nuts), carbohydrates (wholegrains, sweet potatoes, quinoa), fats (healthy oils, avocado, oily fish, nuts), vitamins, minerals and water. These foods have been linked to some disease prevention, such as osteoporosis, high blood pressure, heart disease, diabetes and certain cancers.

If you eat too much, you won't see your body fat reducing, but if you eat too little this can have the same effect. This is because if you are not eating enough calories your body will perceive you to be in a state of famine and hold onto any fat storage (usually around your mid-section) because it doesn't know when the next energy source is coming. Nutrition is unique to each individual and I would always recommend speaking to a nutritional therapist when it comes to optimising your nutrition. The following are general guidelines only that can help kick start your health and fitness lifestyle:

- Eat a wide variety of fruits and vegetables
- Eat whole grains where possible
- Eat lean, healthy protein at every meal
- Include healthy fats
- Cook with healthy oils like avocado oil
- Include fibre (wholegrains, legumes, fruit, vegetables, beans, nuts and seeds) to help fill you up and avoid overeating.
- Eat when you feel hungry and try not to snack between meals.
- Fast overnight (for 12 hours if you can). This allows your blood sugar and insulin to drop and opens up your "longevity" pathways. Your body fat burns preferentially and it helps to control cravings, lower inflammation, and stabilise your energy.

4. EXERCISE

Exercise is, of course, one of the foundational habits, but if you read the above section on making the habit of exercise shorter so it feels easier and you heard yourself saying *"But is 15 minutes of exercise a day really enough?"*, then I want to reassure you that, yes, it is.

Is 15 minutes enough?

Good health is one of, if not THE most important things for our longevity and happiness. Time doesn't need to be your enemy. You can still reap benefits from exercising on a regular basis for 15 minutes a day. First of all, 15 minutes is doable! You CAN easily find, or make, 15 minutes in a day to move your body. I bet you could make the time for something you perceive to be fun, important, or worthwhile, like a night out with friends, watching the new Netflix series, scrolling through your phone/social media, or attending your dental appointments. So why not something that is improving your health?

A 15 minute workout will also help to improve your heart strength and increase your fitness so you are ready for longer workouts. If you are sedentary, you will see your greatest gains from doing short workouts to begin with. The great thing about exercise is that the more you do, the more you want to do!

Building muscle mass is really important as we age. Women, in particular, suffer a decline in muscle mass from the age of 35 and over. Short, intense workouts can target more than one muscle group to increase strength and build more muscle mass.

When you exercise, your body will release chemicals called endorphins. These endorphins trigger a positive feeling in the body and lift your mood. When your mood is lifted, you are more motivated to workout and more pleasant to be around! If you are aware of this change in mood as you exercise, ensure you use it as an intrinsic reward to help embed the habit. Depending on your chosen workout, it can also be fun. If you are doing something similar to the ballet-inspired workout I teach, this is a wonderful opportunity to be 'in the moment'. You have to focus on your body during these workouts, which means you are switching off completely from daily life. It provides a distraction to any ongoing worries you have and so is good for your mental health.

THE 4 TENDENCIES AND HABITS

Understanding how you operate is key to creating new habits. When you shape your habits to suit yourself, you can find success, even when you have failed before. The table below shows how, according to your Tendency, you can best create new habits.

TENDENCY	HABIT	TAKEAWAY
Upholder	• You find keeping habits easier than the other tendencies. • You feel worse if you let yourself off the hook. • You love routine and discipline - this gives you freedom. • Clarity with your chosen process goals is important for you.	Get clarity on your goals and stick to your routine.
Questioner	• You find keeping habits easy provided they are justified. • You need to know that the form of exercise you have chosen is the most efficient and productive way to get fit. • Try different forms of exercise as an experiment - you love to customise. • Be curious about forms of exercise which will help motivate you and find pleasure in learning.	Ensure you can justify the type of exercise you have chosen.
Obliger	• You need outer accountability to create your exercise habit. • Have a friend attend a class with you, or hire a personal trainer or find an accountability buddy. • The key for you is to find the right accountability for you (which we will look at in Chapter 11). • You enjoy the satisfaction of working with others.	You need outer accountability to create an exercise habit.

| Rebel | • You will resist doing exercise if you feel you are being asked or told to do it.
• Strategies that work for other tendencies won't work for you.
• You can embrace a new habit if you view it as a way to express your identity.
• Tie in your habit of exercise to your deep values.
• Reframing techniques can work well for you - "*I can do whatever I want and I want to exercise to improve my health and wellbeing*" as opposed to "*This person expects me to exercise, so I'm not doing it*".
• Rather than scheduling in exercise, keep a record of when classes are and choose to do them when you feel like it.
• Seek out information on the benefits of exercise for you - this helps you to make a decision.
• You are also motivated by a challenge so find personal meaning in pursuing a goal that is difficult, but not impossible. | View exercise as an expression of your identity. |

TIPS TO ENSURE YOU STICK TO YOUR HABITS

Focus on right now

If your plan is to workout daily (even if just for 10 minutes) focus on the immediate future – getting to the end of the workout. Do the job directly in front of you. To help with this, you can use Mel Robbins' "The 5 Second Rule".[6] This rule allows you to beat your brain at its own game and distract it from the ways it's trying to sabotage you, like procrastinating. You will always have an urge to skip your workout. That's ok. You are not a failure for feeling the urge.

Instead, when you feel triggered to procrastinate, count backwards from 5 (5-4-3-2-1) to replace the negative action with something positive like, *"I am going to workout now"*. You know that as soon as you hear that positive message your brain will start to find every excuse under the sun as to why you should skip the workout and not follow through.

For example, if you have got up early to complete a workout and, after putting on your workout gear, you know your brain is going to start telling you to *"wait"* and suggest that *"maybe later would be a better time"*, you need to switch gears. So instead, the moment you hear that internal positive message (*"I am going to workout now"*), start counting backwards from 5. Tell yourself that when you get to 1, you will be on your mat ready to go, or be outside your front door, trainers on and ready to run. Whatever it is you want to do, commit to starting it after the count of 1. Don't wait until you "feel like it". The chances are you are never going to feel like it!

The moment you have an instinct to exercise, push yourself to move within 5 seconds, or your brain will kill it. You have a tiny window of time to take positive action there.

Soon, instead of hesitation, your default mode becomes taking action. This is you being who you want to be and at the same time, developing new neural pathways to create habits so that it gets easier every time to follow through on those positive behaviours.

This method worked really well for a client, Emma, who was struggling to get up in the morning when her alarm went off. She would hit the snooze button at least three times before reluctantly getting out of bed. She felt tired and overwhelmed most of the time, which was not helping her to focus and be productive as a busy lawyer, raising two children. When I told her she was losing about four hours in productivity that day after waking because she was hitting the snooze button, she was very motivated to stop doing it.

How you wake up in the morning impacts your productivity. The snooze button creates a mental state in your brain called sleep inertia. When you go to bed, you sleep in cycles of around 90 minutes all night.[7] Before you wake up in the morning, the sleep cycles stop and your brain wakes up so it can start the day. When the alarm goes off, your brain is ready to start the day. If you snooze, you have made your brain go back into a sleep cycle, which takes another 90 minutes to complete. The trouble is, when the alarm goes off a second time you are only 15 minutes into your sleep cycle. It then takes almost four hours to snap out of that sleep cycle. This leaves you feeling groggy, unable to focus during the day and feeling like you have not had enough sleep. It directly impacts your productivity, alertness, and brain processes for the first four hours of the day.[8]

If you are waking feeling tired, groggy and lacking in energy, what are the chances of you actually completing a workout? Or being productive enough during your day to carve out time for a workout later?

Imagine how good it will feel

This is where you can rehearse past successes (go and read your Evidence Journal for reminders!). Imagine what it will be like when you complete the workout. Tell yourself how good it will feel to be making progress. Breakdown the workout into smaller sections so every section feels good. Once you have completed your warm up, tell yourself, *"I'm a third of the way through now, just the workout and the cool down."* Habits are evidence of success, so make a habit of noticing how you feel.

Be your own cheerleader

While exercising, talk to yourself. Imagine you are your own personal trainer. What would they be saying to you while you were exercising, especially when it starts to become challenging? Tell yourself, *"You can do it"* or, *"This is easy"*, or, *"My body loves exercise"*. These statements are supportive, show self-compassion and are encouraging. Saying, *"Ugh, I have a blister now"*, or *"This is exhausting"* are useful messages coming from your body and definitely worth paying attention to, but they are not necessarily helpful to you at the time. And neither is a statement like *"God, I hate this"*. Yep, I know you have said it!

CHAPTER SUMMARY

- Tiny changes/improvements can have a big impact over time. So small goals can be highly effective in achieving your destination goal.
- Making those small changes, sticking with them and regularly repeating them will turn them into habits you perform automatically - they will become routines.

- The trick is to support the change by having simple cues that trigger the desired action, which will lead to a related immediate reward that you desire.
- If you get it right, then the actions will happen and become habit-forming.
- There are four key foundational habits that will help you to become fitter and healthier - movement (obviously), sleep, stress management and nutrition. The Move, Nourish, Nurture process goals will help you develop these habits.

NEXT STEPS

MY NON-NEGOTIABLES

I suggest you start with no more than three new habits to work on. To help you identify what these habits are, grab a pen and three sheets of paper - one sheet of paper for Move, one for Nourish and one for Nurture. You can write these headings at the top of each sheet. Or, if you prefer, you can start with Move only for now. Nourish and Nurture are going to assist with your Move goal, but in order to avoid over-whelm, selecting one small habit at this stage is absolutely fine.

1. On each sheet of paper draw a cloud, or circle, in the centre.
2. Using the sheets, write your chosen goal (just one for each sheet) inside the cloud.

3. Next, come up with ten or more behaviours that would lead you to your goal. Write each behaviour outside the cloud with arrows pointing toward the cloud. These can be one-time behaviours, or behaviours to be repeated. Be wildly optimistic! If I could wave a magic wand and get you to do any behaviour, what would it be?

4. Put a star by four or five behaviours that you believe would be highly effective in reaching your goal. Think only about the impact of these behaviours, not the feasibility, or practicality of them.

5. Circle any effective behaviours that you can easily get yourself to do (e.g., drink two litres of water a day; get up 15 minutes earlier to exercise). Be realistic. Imagine yourself doing the behaviour in your actual life. Do you feel a little sense of dread when you think about doing it, or do you feel excited about it?

6. Find the behaviours that have both a star and a circle. Those are your non-negotiable process goals.

7. Think of a way to make your non-negotiables a reality in your life. Write down ways that you can make it more obvious, attractive, easy and rewarding.

EXAMPLES OF MY BEHAVIOURS

If my goal was to exercise first thing in the morning, my behaviours might be:

- Set my alarm to go to bed at 9.30pm.
- Arrange my workout clothes next to my bed ready for the morning.
- Decide which workout I will do tomorrow morning and set up my mat and tablet to follow along (if it's an online workout).
- Set an alarm for 6am.
- Complete a bedtime ritual by 10pm and switch the lights out.
- When the alarm goes off at 6am, get out of bed straight away and go to my mat.

The ones I think would have the most impact are setting my alarm to go to bed, setting my alarm to get up early and actually getting up. The alarm setting is easy because it's a one-time behaviour that I can pre-set. I'm not sure how easy getting up at 6am will be, but I will keep it on my list because I will find a way to do this.

8

CRACKING THE CODE

Removing certain habits from your life can be challenging but it's the next step towards achieving your goals, after beginning to create new healthy habits. In this chapter, we will look at the old habits that are sabotaging your efforts to exercise, and preventing you from prioritising your health and wellbeing.

I don't like describing these unwanted behaviours as "bad" habits because they are not necessarily bad and neither are you. At some point in your life, the habits you have developed have served a purpose for you. They made you feel better, or distracted you from uncomfortable thoughts, or feelings. That's why you clung on to them for so long. But they are not helpful any more and don't fit into the lifestyle you want to achieve. Or maybe you just want more effective strategies that don't replace one discomfort with another. We will call them "old" habits, because you are going to be replacing them with "new", healthy habits.

UNDERSTANDING YOUR "OLD" HABITS

On most occasions, old habits are a way of dealing with stress and boredom. Everything from biting your nails, to drinking every weekend, to dipping into the treat box after meals, to wasting time browsing the internet can be a simple response to stress and boredom. When you feel stress, you want to push that feeling away and distract yourself as quickly as possible. Of course there are stressful situations that cannot be avoided in life but it's important to remember that there is never the "perfect" time to take yourself through a period of change and you have to face some degree of discomfort.

Sometimes, there could be certain beliefs or reasons that are behind the old habits. There might be a fear, an event, tiredness, or a limiting belief that is causing you to hold on to something that is bad for you. If you are a worrier, the rumination can leave you feeling emotionally exhausted and less able to deal with the discomfort of change head on.

The frustrating part is that these old habits, which are fairly entrenched in most cases, can be hard to change. This is because often, these old habits are pleasure-based habits. Enjoyable behaviours prompt your brain to release dopamine (the feel good hormone). When you are repeating a behaviour over and over again and dopamine is present when you're doing it, this strengthens the habit even more. And when you're not doing the behaviour, dopamine creates the craving to do it again.

These behaviours can become hardwired in our brains and even when we are trying hard to resist, the brain's reward centre keeps us craving it. The good news is, with practice, we can change these patterns of behaviour towards long-term goals, creating new neural pathways that help create "good" habits for achieving those goals.

But we must remember, there's no single effective way to break old habits. It's not a one size fits all approach and we need to take into consideration our personal tendencies and the strategies that will work best for us as unique individuals.

WHAT DOESN'T WORK

So many of my clients describe *"falling off the wagon"*, or needing to *"get back on track"* with their healthy habits. Sometimes this happens because of negative self-talk that has been triggered by an event or person, or sometimes it's coming back from holiday and realising several weeks later that they're still in holiday mode. Or often, it's just that they are tired, or they forgot they were meant to be changing their behaviour because it's been a busy week and they are on autopilot.

What's important is that you start to identify what isn't working for you. Those approaches you always seem to go back to even though they have never really worked for you in the first place. For example, weight loss shakes, or medical liquid diets, that work over the 12-16 week period but aren't sustainable over the long-term. Or the heavy cardio and minimal calories approach to weight loss that leaves you feeling exhausted. These are short-term options that mean you have to "start again" to maintain your goal. And the pattern repeats. They are useful so long as they last, but are only necessary because the way you "normally" live, exercise, eat etc., does not result in you having the health/fitness/body you want all the time. Far better to make smaller and more realistic changes, that you can sustain long-term, so that you don't need quick fixes.

Noticing your patterns is vital for your motivation to exercise. If you are setting yourself up to fail, this will lead to negative self-talk about how useless and weak you are. You are then likely to repeat the old behaviour, leading to weight gain/ loss of muscle tone, which means you sign up for the liquid diet again, or the fad fitness programme.

What is triggering your old habits? Does one glass of wine in an evening lead to another glass, which leads to more snacking, a late night and tiredness, which means you hit the snooze button the next morning instead of getting up and working out? Does saying "*yes*" to another friend in need lead to you feeling overwhelmed and exhausted with no time or energy to exercise? Does having your phone with you at all times lead to browsing the internet when you are bored, wasting 20 minutes or more when you could be prepping some healthy food or going out for a walk in nature or actually going to sleep earlier?

I'm not a fan of the expressions *"falling off the wagon"* or *"getting back on track"* when it comes to your healthy habits. They imply you have completely removed yourself from the wagon, or track. You see only two options, either you are on, or off the wagon. If you are on, you are 100% committed to your exercise regime and if you are off, you are not working out at all.

This all-or-nothing thinking has GOT to go. This *does not* mean throwing in the towel on health. It means understanding that health is a journey. It means realising that there are a lot of options in between doing nothing at all and doing everything perfectly. Instead of seeing yourself flying through the air off that wagon and landing in a ditch each time you perceive yourself as failing, choose to see yourself staying seated on the wagon (or a more fancy vehicle perhaps!). Accept that, occasionally, your chosen vehicle slows down while you gather your resources, or sometimes it gets a little rocky over turbulent terrain. When things get really bad, your control over the steering may suffer. But in-between these hiccups, your journey runs smoothly.

You probably can't do everything perfectly and sustain your healthy habits, but you can always do something.

WHICH HABITS DO YOU WANT TO STOP?

We know from previous chapters that the most important areas for consideration (in addition to exercise) when it comes to optimising our health, are sleep, nutrition (including hydration) and reducing stress. When we have control over these areas, we are placing ourselves in a much better position to be motivated to exercise. So, if you are lacking in quality sleep, eating junk food, and experiencing high levels of stress, there will be a number of habits that are contributing to these unwanted behaviours, which you can now begin to remove.

You must be clear on which habits you want to stop. They are usually the ones that are not serving you well, or helping you towards achieving your goal. But just as when you are crafting your goals, you need to be specific when it comes to identifying the old habit you want to stop.

If you are saying *"I want to stop eating junk food"*, this might sound specific to you, but it is not. This is the general habit, which comprises a tangle of habits. If you imagine this general habit as a knot, you need to focus on untangling it. There will be habits, or tangles, that require some work in order to make progress with the general habit, or knot. For example, the tangles that make up the knot might be: putting sugar in your tea, eating crisps while you watch TV in the evening, always having something sweet after a meal, snacking on the treats brought into the office, picking on your children's food, drinking fizzy drinks with lunch, snacking on a chocolate bar to get over the 4pm afternoon slump, or making sandwiches with white bread and processed meat. These are the specific habits to work on so you can untangle that knot.

To help identify the patterns involved for each of your old habits, spend a few days tracking each habit to see whether they follow any patterns. Record things like:

- Where does the habitual behaviour happen?
- What time of day?
- How do you feel when it happens?
- Are other people involved?
- Does it happen right after, or as part of, something else?

Let's say you want to stop staying up past midnight so you can rise earlier and workout. After a few days of tracking your behaviour, you may realise you tend to stay up later if you start watching TV, or chatting with friends after dinner, or checking your emails or social media when relaxing before bed. But you go to bed earlier if you read, or take a walk.

This pattern of staying up late is quite common for busy women with demanding families. "Revenge bedtime procrastination" refers to a phenomenon of wanting more "me" time at the end of the day. You put off going to bed early in order to do the things you have been unable to do during the day because of lack of any time to yourself. This could either be work, or pleasure - you just want some space to focus on you! When my children were smaller, I frequently said to my husband in the evenings *"I just need some time to myself"*, which inevitably meant I was heading to bed late after catching up with work and waking exhausted and repeating the same pattern the following day, but even less effectively, because I was too tired to do anything particularly constructive during the day.

Having clarity over your patterns of behaviour means that you can start to make different decisions. You can decide to stop watching TV and turn off your phone by 9pm on weeknights. You can replace this with an evening bedtime routine that is relaxing and more conducive to a good night's sleep. Removing the trigger - e.g. watching TV - makes it harder to carry out the routine of staying up too late.

Other habits that I see compromising women's health are:

- Worrying about the future and harbouring regrets from the past, which causes stress and low mood;
- Obsessing over appearance, which is damaging to mental health and can lead to damage to physical health if extreme diets, yo-yo dieting, or cosmetic surgery are involved;
- Putting themselves last and running themselves into the ground.

What other habits do you have that are sabotaging your efforts to lead a healthy, happy life? You don't need to start removing them all at once, but it is important to identify them, so you can get a clearer picture of your patterns and how they interrelate.

WHY DO YOU WANT TO STOP THEM?

Take a few minutes to consider why you want to break your old habit and any benefits you see resulting from the change. It is likely to be easier to change your behaviour when the change you want to make is valuable, or beneficial to you. Is the reason for removal of the habit associated with improving your mental, physical, or emotional wellbeing? What will be the impact on your life if you are able to remove this old habit? Or, is your reason connected to someone else? Do you want to remove this habit so you are able to spend more quality time with your family?

Habits tend to form much more quickly if you have a strong positive emotion connected to the behaviour and the same works in the reverse. If you have a strong negative emotion connected to the behaviour, it will be much easier to remove it from your life. Focus on the importance to you of removing the habit and not on why you think you "should" remove it.

HOW DO YOU STOP?

We know from the previous chapter that there are four elements to a habit - a cue, a craving, a response, and a reward.

A cue triggers the brain to start the desired behaviour. The craving is the desire for change. The response is the actual habit, action or behaviour and the reward is the end goal that satisfies the craving and tells us which actions are worth remembering.

Just as you can make a habit easier to adopt by altering any of these four components, you can do the same to stop a behaviour. To create a new habit we looked at strategies to make the habits obvious, attractive, easy and satisfying. With old habits that we want to stop, we need to do the reverse. We need to make them:

1. Invisible,
2. Unattractive,
3. Difficult, and
4. Unsatisfying.

Some of this relies on you changing your environment, which we will look at in chapter 10, but let's take a deeper dive here.

1. MAKE IT INVISIBLE

To make a habit invisible you can remove it altogether, avoid it, or ignore it. For example, if you want to stop checking your phone when you get into bed at night, you could turn off your phone, put it on do not disturb mode, or turn off any notifications for social media apps. You could also leave your phone in another room entirely. If you are snacking on Doritos each evening, get rid of any packets already in your house and stop buying them (don't even walk down the crisp aisle in the supermarket). Let your family know what you are doing, so they don't bring any packets into the house unwittingly.

If you can't remove the cue, or trigger, you can still avoid it. Let's say you want to stop grabbing a pastry with your morning coffee on the way to work, you could stop going to the coffee shop and make a coffee at home with your breakfast before leaving the house.

Your final option is to ignore the trigger altogether, but this is more challenging because it involves willpower and requires extra effort. You will need to recruit other strategies to ignore the trigger, such as self-compassion, or paying closer attention to your identity, which we will look at in the next chapter.

2. MAKE IT UNATTRACTIVE

This is when revisiting your goals, values, and beliefs is important. To make an old habit unattractive, you need to reframe your mindset and ask yourself whether it is in alignment with how you want to live your life. Instead of thinking about how bad a habit is for you, think of all the benefits of not doing it.

Avoid saying, *"I don't want to eat junk food"* as this will activate a part of your brain that just hears "junk food" and makes you crave it. The subconscious brain cannot process the word "don't", so when you don't want to think about something, you do. Instead, reframe it by saying *"I want to be healthy and fit"*. Quitting junk food will take you towards this goal.

3. MAKE IT HARDER

To make a habit harder, you make it inconvenient by increasing the time it requires, the money it requires, the physical and mental effort, and making it conflict with important routines.

Making habits inconvenient helps us stick to our good habits. For example, leaving the phone in another room increases the number of steps you have to take to scroll through Facebook. You have to get up, walk to another room, find the phone, walk back and then start scrolling, rather than simply picking up the phone at your desk and mindlessly scrolling out of habit because you are bored.

4. MAKE IT UNSATISFYING

Succeeding with this step is about making the punishment for completing your old habit worse than the pleasure you get from doing it. Life is a game of incentives and the biggest motivators are the desire for pleasure and the avoidance of pain.

To create pain associated with your old habit, an accountability partner can work really well. We care deeply about what others think of us and we do not want others to have a lesser opinion of us. If you are trying to quit sugar, you will feel the pressure to quit if you are reporting to someone each day about the last time you had a chocolate bar or a bowl of ice-cream. The guilt of admitting defeat and hurting your ego may be the only force powerful enough to overcome the dopamine hit from sneaking a sugar fix in on your afternoon break or late at night.

OTHER STRATEGIES

Substitute an old habit with a new one

You need to have a plan ahead of time when you start to feel stressed, or bored, which prompts the old habit you are trying to ditch. We know that your old habits are there for a reason and have served you in the past, so trying to remove them entirely or just "stop doing it" does not always work for everyone. Instead, substitute the old habit for something new. If your old habit is to browse the internet when you get bored working, substitute this browsing with a stretch, or get up from your desk and take a short walk around the garden or office.

It's better to replace your bad habits with a healthier behaviour that addresses that same need. So, if you are prone to eating when you feel stressed, to meet this same need, try taking some deep breaths to calm yourself down. Or how about substituting it with curiosity about why you are having that craving in the first place, and what it feels like in your body and your mind? Creating time and space in the moment allows you to really assess what is going on and ask yourself, *"Am I actually hungry?"* If the answer is "no", ask yourself what else is going on. This gives you the opportunity to realise that you are stressed and discover what has triggered that stress response. When you have this information, you are in a far better position to deal with the source of the stress, rather than ruminating after giving into the old habit and in turn, feeling anxious and disappointed.

Distract yourself

Distraction works best when it involves physical activity like cleaning, walking, gardening, emptying the dishwasher, playing with your child, or tidying your desk. Research shows that with active distraction, urges usually subside within about fifteen minutes. So the next time you have the urge to get up from your desk to grab a biscuit (out of habit rather than hunger), tell yourself you will wait fifteen minutes and then leave your desk. The delay may mean you get absorbed in doing something different and you forget about your craving completely.

Use the word "but"

Use the word "but" to overcome negative self–talk. When you slip up and revert to your old habits, it's easy to judge yourself for not making a different decision. Each time you find yourself being mean and admonishing yourself for yet another mistake, finish the sentence with "but":

- *"I'm out of shape, but I could be in shape in a few months' time."*
- *"I'm so bad at running, but I'm working to develop this skill."*
- *"I'm a failure, but everybody fails sometimes."*

Get support

As we will see in chapter 11, surrounding yourself with like-minded women, who are already working towards similar goals and have succeeded in changing their habits and behaviours, will give you the necessary encouragement and support your need to do the same.

Keeping good habits has its cost - time, money, pleasures - but not keeping good habits also has its cost. Which cost do you want to pay?

YOUR TENDENCY AND BREAKING OLD HABITS

By better understanding your reasons for doing things according to your Tendency, you can start to be more aware of how some of your old habits may have formed and what you can do now to break them.

TENDENCY	OLD HABIT	TAKEAWAY
Upholder	• Your inner expectations help you to resist any excuses not to exercise. • You find resisting old habits easier than other tendencies. • Clarity over why you are ditching your old habits is important for you.	Find clarity over why you are ditching your old habits.
Questioner	• You feel greater pressure from your own inner expectations to resist excuses not to exercise. • Find ways to make your old habits unjustifiable. • Know that your old habits are not an efficient or productive way to get fit.	See your old habits as inefficient and unproductive so you can justify ditching them.
Obliger	• You struggle against the temptations of excuses not to exercise. • You need accountability to support you in ditching old habits. • You are sometimes at risk of looking for ways to get around having any external accountability, because you know that's what supports you in abstaining from old habits.	Find external accountability to help you ditch your old habits.
Rebel	• You don't make excuses to justify doing what you want. • You need to tie in removing old habits with your deep core values. • Seek out information on the downside to following your old habits to help you decide what to do. • See resisting old habits as an expression of your identity.	See resisting old habits as an expression of your identity and focus on the downside of continuing with them.

CHAPTER SUMMARY

- As well as starting to create new, healthy habits, it's necessary to remove existing habits that have been unhelpful in achieving your health and fitness goals.
- There's no single simple solution to breaking "bad" habits - you need to find the best way for you.
- But first, you need to identify clearly what the habits are that you want/need to break and what is triggering them so that you can focus on starting to change them.
- Accept that this will take time and you won't always succeed perfectly. Health is a journey - there are smooth bits and bumpy bits and everything in between. There are lots of options between doing nothing to get there and doing everything perfectly.
- There may be general habits you want to stop - e.g. eating junk food. That general habit will be made up of a tangle of other behaviors and habits. Identify what they are so you can start unpicking them, one by one - which will be far more manageable than trying to deal with them all at once.
- Focus on the importance to you of removing the habit and the benefits of doing so. This will help you see the emotional connection to the habit that will make it easier to overcome.
- Make the unwanted habits harder to continue - by making it: invisible (i.e. removing the cue); unattractive (focus on the benefits of <u>not</u> doing it);

harder (by making it inconvenient); and unsatisfying (by creating "pain" by doing it or making the punishment worse than the pleasure you get from it).

- Also, consider and plan other tools you will use to help you when you find yourself craving the old/bad habit - identify a substitute healthy behaviour next time (or whenever) the relevant cue occurs, which addresses the same need.

- Think about how you can distract yourself from doing the bad behaviour until the desire subsides - if you can do this for 15 minutes, you will probably avoid the bad behaviour.

- Don't judge yourself harshly if you slip up - if you berate yourself for doing so, finish the sentence with "*but…*".

NEXT STEPS

1. MY OLD HABITS

I suggest you start with no more than three old habits. Grab a pen and three sheets of paper - one sheet for each of your old habits. If you only have one or two old habits, that's great! You won't need all three sheets. If you have more than three old habits, choose the three you would most like to stop.

1. On each sheet of paper draw a cloud in the centre.
2. Write your general old habit (one for each sheet) inside the cloud.

3. Write down <u>at</u> <u>least</u> ten specific habits around the cloud that lead to the general habit inside the cloud. This may require some imagination.

4. Look over your specific old habits and choose two or three of the easiest to resolve.

5. For each of your chosen three habits, decide how you can make the habit invisible, unattractive, difficult and/or unsatisfying. You can use the table below to record this.

An example: if I wanted to stop eating too much junk food (general habit to place inside the cloud) my specific habits might be:

- Eating chocolate on the commute home from work.
- Making a sandwich of white bread and processed meat.
- Eating crisps while I watch TV in the evening.
- Drinking a glass of wine as soon as I stop work/put the kids to bed.
- Putting sugar in my tea.
- Drinking carbonated drinks every day at lunch.
- Eating 3 slices of pizza for lunch.
- Eating a cookie in my break each morning.

MY OLD HABIT	HOW I CAN MAKE THEM INVISIBLE, UNATTRACTIVE, DIFFICULT, OR UNSATISFYING
1.	
2.	
3.	

2. WHAT'S THE COST?

Looking at your chosen old habits from above, I want you to start projecting into the future to bring about a sense of urgency with your habits. To do this, start by considering what life might look like if you don't make any changes to your current lifestyle and behaviours. This will help to challenge any *"I'll start exercising when life calms down"* thinking.

Choose a specific future date, say in six- or 12-months' time, and start writing down all the words and sentences describing how you think things will look across your life if you don't manage to make the changes you'd like to make. You can write them in the table below, or use a spider diagram, or map. Whatever helps organise this information in a logical way for your brain. I personally love spider diagrams because my brain works best with that visual presentation. Make sure you are including statements on how you will feel, what you will see and hear and what you will be saying to yourself. Try to visualise your future self as clearly as possible.

I have done this exercise with many clients. Here are some of the things that came up for them:

- Nothing changes and I allow depression to take over. Plus, I stay flabbier and less strong than I need to be.
- Health problems and/or feeling depressed.
- I worry that my anxiety would worsen and my focus and enthusiasm would dwindle further. I want to be a mum that has fun and a woman who loves life rather than simply surviving.
- Losing my spirit/shine, probably becoming sicker.
- To be honest, I don't even want to think about it. I still believe that one day, I will turn my life to normal without stress eating, working crazy hours etc.
- I won't have fully achieved my ambitions in life, my knee may deteriorate if I don't stay active, my mental health may suffer.
- Those risk factors, lack of sleep = lack of energy, lapse in concentration and focus. The thought of being in an 'at risk' bracket scares me as I get older. I want to be the best version of me that I can be.

These are a fraction of the very honest and real responses I received from women to this question, expressing fear and concern for their futures. They are women in their 40s and beyond who are just like you and me. They are not lazy, lacking in willpower, or hopeless cases. They are living busy lives and at the time of writing, had not yet found the right personal strategies.

When you have your list, or diagram, rate out of ten how important each of these things is to you personally (10 being very important and 1 being not that important). Remember, you are not scoring these words based on what you think "should" be most important, but on what is personally important to you.

OLD HABIT	WHAT LIFE WILL LOOK LIKE IF IT CONTINUES

3. WHAT WILL TRIP ME UP?

Repeat the same exercise as above (in the table below, or a spider diagram), but this time, write down what it is that generally causes you to feel stress, or worry, or become overwhelmed and tired, or start with the negative self-talk. This will help you to identify the causes, or triggers, for your unwanted behaviours.

OLD HABIT	WHAT WILL TRIP ME UP?

9

EXERCISE IDENTITY

I grew up in a four-bedroom detached house, on the coast of North Wales. Like everyone else, my childhood was filled with daily learnings and constant reminders of my social identity. I was a painfully shy child, daughter of a bank manager and a stay-at-home mum, a red-head, who went to state school, who was ballet-obsessed and adored horse-riding. I was sporty, but also a complete bookworm. I was clever and did well at school, but had quite a turbulent school life as a sensitive child. Each of these layers defined who I was. These layers also defined my social group - who I could call my own because of our collective identity. In this book, I refer to your social group as your "tribe" and we will look at this in more detail in Chapter 11.

My mother was university educated and the expectation was that my brother and I would tread that same path. We watched many televised sports in my house growing up. My

Nana had played tennis for Wales, my mum was in the (men's) squash league and my father had been a talented cross country runner. My father never missed a televised Liverpool football match, and was an avid watcher of snooker, boxing, and cricket. Wimbledon tennis was also a firm fixture in our house. Over the years, I attended multiple ballet performances with my mum and Auntie Ethel (who wasn't really my auntie and must have been well into her 80s on these theatre trips). My brother was a keen athlete and rugby player.

I don't recall ever being pushed into physical activity. It was a normal part of our lives. It was who we were. We knew where we belonged and who our tribe was. We knew our likes and dislikes, what our capabilities were and the environments in which we felt accepted.

This was my identity, based on my social and cultural upbringing.

WHAT IS IDENTITY?

The word identity was originally derived from the Latin words *essentitas*, which means *being* (or essence), and *identidem*, which means *repeatedly*. Your identity is literally your "repeated beingness". Our identity emerges from our habits.

We are not born with pre-set beliefs. All of them are learned and conditioned through our childhood experiences (coupled with certain genetic predispositions). These sets of qualities and beliefs are what make one person different from another.

How we each view ourselves combined with our social environment is what shapes our identity. We want to be with similar people, who have similar interests and outlooks on life. We pick the language, appearance and behaviours of our tribe and we adopt them. We also have a clear understanding of who is *not* in our tribe.

Of course, you are not a child anymore and your identity can shift over time. In the long run, if you are struggling to commit to your healthy habits, this could be because your self-image is getting in the way. This is why it's not a good idea to get too attached to one version of your identity. In order for us to progress with our lives, sometimes we have to unlearn, or edit our beliefs, and to upgrade our identity. It certainly wouldn't be helpful for me to keep believing I was the shy person I was growing up. It would have stopped me doing half the things I now do in my life and business.

Identity is a highly personal and multi-dimensional component of how we view ourselves. Fitness, or exercise, is just one part of that identity.

WHAT IS EXERCISE IDENTITY?

Exercise identity is one of the largest psychological influences of exercise.[1] In other words, if you have a strong exercise identity, you are far more likely to be exercising on a consistent basis.

What does your exercise identity look like? Try answering the following questions:

- Do you consider yourself to be an active, or physically fit person?
- Are you a frequent exerciser?
- Do you associate yourself with doing a particular kind of sport or exercise?
- Would you describe yourself this way to others?

Your answers to the above questions are at the centre of whether or not you have a strong exercise identity. These questions help you to determine your exercise identity, which in turn determines how you are likely to spend your free time.

Exercise identity is the extent to which you believe that exercise is an important component of who you are as a person. It defines your self-concept as an exerciser. People who are more likely to develop an exercise identity are the people who view exercise as necessary, enjoyable, who are motivated to exercise and who see themselves as capable of doing so.

What contributes to your exercise identity?

As you can see from my example above, our social and cultural norms have a big influence on our exercise identity. Your age, gender identity and social/cultural acceptance and attractiveness all have a role to play here. Have you ever wondered whether you are too old, or too young, to be taking part in a particular exercise regime? You may have questioned whether you are capable of doing so. As a woman, you may have felt that prioritising yourself over others causes conflict with your accepted role as a nurturer. Gender roles may also have influenced your likes and dislikes of particular forms of exercise (or any exercise!).

You may be wondering how social / cultural acceptance and attractiveness play a part here too. The answer is that all these identities have a direct impact on our expectations of appropriateness - whether we think the particular exercise regime is suitable, or proper, in the circumstances. This in turn influences (1) your confidence to exercise, and (2) how important exercise is to you.

Lack of confidence plays a part

Lack of confidence in exercising can be an issue for some women. There may be a fear of being judged (too old/young/large/small/fit/unfit etc.), or not fitting in (not wearing the right clothes, comparing yourself to others who you perceive to be fitter, thinner, or healthier). There could be issues with physical self-image and the ability to understand what is required, how to do it, and the best way to go about achieving your goal.

Lack of confidence can also impact your enjoyment of exercise and can be a barrier to exercising for women. But confidence is a choice and something you can grow. It is not something we are born with, or without. You may feel that when it comes to exercise, it is not reasonable for you to feel confident. If your mind has been telling you that you are hopeless, have no willpower and have two left feet, you can see why this might be the case. Adopting a new identity can help you to change who you are being, not just what you are doing.

Your confidence in exercising also impacts how you view the importance of exercising (which we know is also influenced by social and cultural norms). It could affect how seriously you take your health and your perception of your current level of activity. If you don't feel confident with exercise, you are likely to regard it as low on your list of priorities, telling yourself you are active enough.[2]

This lack of confidence to exercise, coupled with the low perceived importance of exercise, can impact your willingness to overcome pre-existing social or cultural identities in order to exercise.

As you have seen from previous chapters, all these factors will lead to specific beliefs about exercise, which then reinforce the habits that are required to maintain that identity. It's a feedback loop. The beliefs feed into the habits, which in turn feed into the identity, which means we exercise more frequently, which once again strengthens our identity. For example, one study indicated that people believe an exercise identity is maintained by the prioritising of exercise, exercising for a purpose, exercising consistently, and exercising with a particular frequency, duration, and intensity.[3]

Fitness identity is the key to working out more frequently with better results. With a strong fitness identity, you are more likely to make greater plans, or goals, for your exercise than people with low, or no, fitness identity.[4] As you can see from my childhood experiences, past experiences with exercise contribute in helping to build an exercise identity.[5] On the flip side, past experiences can also hinder this process if the experience has been a negative one.

But the good news is, the act of exercising itself helps to build your fitness identity, and you can also begin to develop and upgrade your identity. You can start your exercise journey with whichever side is easier for you - exercising, or building your exercise identity. But the more you exercise, and the more it becomes part of your life, the stronger your exercise identity will become, which will reinforce your desire to exercise and to do it.

With a strong exercise identity you are also more likely to be motivated to exercise for the right reasons - enjoyment, or living in alignment with your values - rather than from guilt, peer pressure, fear, or a negative body image. In chapter 3, we talked about how motivating yourself to exercise is usually done in one of two ways: creating anxiety, or imagining a positive experience. With a greater exercise identity, you will find it much easier to imagine a positive experience when exercising.

Using discomfort to your advantage

I know from experience that women with a strong exercise identity feel uncomfortable when they don't workout regularly. This discomfort is enough motivation to get moving again. There is no need to reflect on your values, beliefs, habits, strategies etc. It's the fitness identity itself that motivates you to move again.

In May 2022, I was bed bound for nearly three weeks following ankle surgery. Once the pain was manageable, I briefly enjoyed the rest and the break from doing all the cooking and other household chores. It gave me time to be more present and get perspective on life. However, this novelty soon wore off and I started to become frustrated at not being able to move around. Whilst some of this was down to lack of independence and wanting to just get on with things and do them my way (control freak), a large part of this frustration was my inability to move in the way I am used to doing.

My clients report the same thing. Once they have established a daily habit of exercise, when they have a break from it (for a holiday, or because life simply gets in the way for a period of time), they find themselves feeling restless and keen to get back to their workout routine.

Kate is a great example of this. On a recent sailing holiday, she really missed her ballet workouts. Her and her friend walked around six miles every day when they got to land so they could stretch their legs, but Kate noticed that it's her ballet workouts that get her up early in the morning and moving. They help her prepare mentally and physically for her day. While she was sailing, she really missed that time. Her motivation to get back to it was because she didn't want to lose the flexibility and strength she had built up. She describes herself as *"always wanting to improve my capabilities...basically future-proofing for my old age!"*.

Gill says she works on *"remembering"* that exercise is a necessity. If she misses her workouts, she knows her back will play up and how debilitating this can be. She says, *"I miss the feeling of being on the 'leaner' side. I benefit from the endorphins. It's an opportunity to 'check in' with my physical body. Otherwise I can live too much in my head / my to-do list / my fast-paced natural default mode with my poor body having to keep up. If I don't make time for my body, it sends me increasingly loud signals and will physically ground me if I don't listen"*. When she hasn't worked out, she misses the discipline, the routine, the time for herself. *"For me, it's not sustainable to not move and stretch and exercise"*.

Ida describes it beautifully. When she hasn't exercised, in order to get back into it she *"digs into memories of how my body feels when I exercise every day. And these are good memories of a body which feels like well-cut clothes. I can move it in every direction I want. The next morning I am back on my routine"*.

To get to this place of experiencing discomfort as motivation to workout, you need to build a strong exercise identity and this is done through developing new habits. It's important to repeat the right behaviours, over and over again, until you *are* those behaviours and have them weaved into your lifestyle.

CHANGING YOUR BEHAVIOUR

When we begin to consider how to embark on this habit journey to develop or upgrade our exercise identity, it can feel a little daunting. So, let's break that down now, so you can see a clear path forwards.

In his book, Atomic Habits, James Clear sets out the three levels of behaviour change:[6]

Changing your outcomes - this level is focused on your goals: losing weight, strengthening your body, or increasing your flexibility. In other words, this is concerned with what you *get*.

1. **Changing your processes** - this level is focused on changing your habits and strategies: implementing a new regime at the gym, following a new online programme, finding an accountability buddy. This level is concerned with what you *do*.
2. **Changing your identity** - this is the deepest level and is concerned with changing your beliefs, your self-image, your judgements about yourself and your biases. This level is about what you *believe*.

Rightly so, we need to establish our goals so we have something to work towards. But as I explained in the previous chapter, our focus shouldn't be on what we *want* to achieve. We need to emotionally let go of the results once we have set ourselves a target. Instead, we can build identity-based habits and focus on *who* we wish to become.

If you have ever set a weight loss goal, you may never have considered identity change when you set out to reach your goal. You will have been thinking about becoming thinner (the outcome / destination goal) and sticking to a diet to achieve this goal (the process goals). This is a great start, but there is a missing piece - the beliefs that drive your actions. If you never shift the way you look at yourself, you may never realise that your old identity can sabotage your new plans for change.

What you need to do is focus on the identity-based habits that will shape and strengthen your new identity.

HABITS ARE THE PATH TO A NEW IDENTITY

Your habits contribute most of the evidence that shapes your identity. You might start a behaviour because you are motivated to do so, but the only reason you will stick with one is because it has become part of your identity, part of who you are. Shifting the belief behind the behaviour will help you to stick to long-term behaviours so that they become habits.

The goal is not to exercise, the goal is to become an exerciser.

When you are able to shift your mindset this way, you are no longer seeking behaviour change, you are simply being the person you already believe yourself to be.

But what if you have deep-seated beliefs that hinder your progress? Like, *"I'm not a morning person, so I can't workout then"*, or *"I'm really unfit"*, or *"I'm hopeless at sticking to an exercise plan"*. Do you recall the behaviour patterns from Chapter 4? The Quitter, the Bull in a china shop, Ostrich etc.? There may be stories you are telling yourself about your fitness.

These types of beliefs can impact your ability to change. The deeper these beliefs are rooted - perhaps from childhood when you never got picked for the school sports teams - the harder they are to change. But it's not impossible and it's important we make these slow changes, no matter how uncomfortable they seem, if ultimately, we want to live a happier, healthier life.

I want you to remember that you are not stuck in your behaviours forever. They do not define you. They are temporary and we have the ability to change them. Just because you are telling yourself you are hopeless and lazy does not mean you are actually hopeless and lazy (even if you haven't exercised for weeks!). If you had to, I'm sure you could list numerous examples of situations where you were successful, energised and active in your attempts to achieve a particular goal. It's just that when it comes to exercise, you may be holding onto an old story, perhaps from your childhood, and your patterns of behaviour are on repeat because you have not changed the channel. Despite our best efforts, when we are having a bad day, it is so easy to fall back into old behaviours.

Changing identity does not mean that you are about to overhaul your entire lifestyle overnight. That doesn't work and is not sustainable. The process of habit change is incremental. We take small, manageable steps on a daily basis, reinforcing the behaviours of the person we wish to become. We want to see evidence every day of this new identity to demonstrate to ourselves that we are making a meaningful difference to our life.

Clear describes this two-step process as follows:

1. Decide on the type of person you want to be.
2. Prove it to yourself with small wins.

You have already looked at your core values when it comes to exercise. Revisit those now and consider what you want to stand for. Who do you wish to become?

If you are finding this tricky, start with your goal. What is your destination goal - the results you ultimately want to achieve through exercise? Let's say it's to strengthen and tone your body. Now ask yourself, *"Who is the type of woman that could gain a strong, toned body?"* It's probably someone who is consistent with their exercise and knows what exercise they need to do to achieve this outcome.

Sometimes it can help to think of yourself in the third person. For example, I can think of the "now" Sarah (married, aged 45, running a business, busy, with two children) and the "future" Sarah (retired, children left home, travelling the world, more time on my hands!). The "now" Sarah is the client and the future me is the personal trainer telling the "now" Sarah what she needs to do. The "now" Sarah may not be exercising regularly, may have insecurities about the way her body looks, or lack confidence in her ability to exercise and make real change. When I go about my day and I'm faced with multiple decisions at every turn that can impact on my habits, I can ask myself, *"What would future Sarah say?"* Or *"What would a healthy woman do?"* My goal is to live a long and healthy life. I can clearly envisage the healthy 70 plus year old that I want to be in my future. It is that woman that gets me up in the morning to workout and steers me away from (too much) chocolate.

My focus is on identity-based habits. My habits shape my identity and my identity shapes my habits. To consistently drive this "feedback loop" and feed into strengthening your fitness identity and building healthy habits, we must focus on our values, principles, and identity, rather than the results. The results will come - they are the side effect of creating the right habits.

And the good news is you don't need to be working out for hours on end every day to upgrade your fitness identity. Yet again, consistency is key, not the duration, or intensity of your workout. Simply walking, or upping the amount of physical activity you include in your day (like climbing the stairs rather than taking the lift, or cycling to a friend's house, rather than driving) will, in time, allow you to see yourself as an exerciser.

REFRAMING YOUR IDENTITY

We know that our minds do not distinguish between what we see in front of us (reality) and what we imagine in our minds. It is all just pictures. Whatever we think about, our unconscious mind will endeavour to create. So, if you think doom and gloom all the time, don't be the slightest bit surprised if that is the way your life is turning out. It is the same with exercise. If you view it as hard work, it will be. Changing the way you view exercise and how it makes you feel is critical to your success and building up your fitness identity.

Imagine how it would feel to choose to go out for your daily walk instead of skipping it so you could catch up on your emails. Prioritising your walk despite your busy schedule means you are identifying as someone who exercises, who is putting their health and wellbeing first.

Visualisation, or mental rehearsal, is a really powerful way to help you to achieve your goals. It is what top athletes use to realise their dreams with a single image. Think of the 100m sprint runner. You see them at the start line at the Olympics, staring down the track with complete focus. They are mentally rehearsing their race, stretching well while waiting for the race to begin. Getting down to the blocks, waiting for the start gun, swiftly moving off the blocks into their stride and how it feels to effortlessly glide down the field at the front.

Sport psychology research rarely focuses exclusively on goal-based images, but instead, the process of achieving a goal.[7] This is because the outcome-based goals are least often used by athletes. They are focusing on the process goals, what they need to do to achieve the outcome. Who they need to be and what they need to be doing in the moment.[8]

And this works for non-athletes too! Research has shown that imagining yourself in the future as physically fit helped retirees gain a stronger physical activity identity one month later.[9]

The more pride you have in your fitness identity, the more motivated you will be to maintain the habits associated with it. For example, if you are really proud of your toned, slim arms and shoulders, you are far more likely to maintain a habit of body weight training, or weight lifting, to maintain the shape of your arms.

HOW IDENTITY AFFECTS THE TENDENCIES

Understanding identity is key for all Tendencies when it comes to exercise but especially so for a Rebel. The table below highlights how each Tendency can benefit from a deeper understanding of the importance of identity to shape your exercise habit.

TENDENCY	IDENTITY	TAKEAWAY
Upholder	• If you have a strong fitness identity this motivates you to stick to your healthy habits. • Don't get too caught up in the past and keep moving forwards.	Keep doing what works for you.
Questioner	• Knowing your fitness identity helps you to tweak your habits to suit your particular character. • A strong fitness identity will help motivate you to stick to your healthy habits.	Tweak your habits to suit your identity.
Obliger	• Telling others about a decision to alter an aspect of your identity can help you stick to your habits. • Remaining part of the group is crucial to maintaining your habits. • Friendship and community help you to embed a new identity.	Tell others about your new identity.
Rebel	• You need to tie your habits to your identity. • You can embrace a habit if you view it as a way to express your identity - to be authentic to yourself. • If you respect yourself, you will want to take care of yourself.	Tie your habit of exercise to your identity.

In chapter 11, we will talk about your social environment and how your identity becomes linked to those around you. The shared identity begins to reinforce your personal identity.

CHAPTER SUMMARY

- How you view yourself - your identity - has a huge input on your behaviour.
- But we all do change and are capable of changing over time in response to our environment, circumstances and desires.
- Your fitness and aptitude for exercise is one part of your identity.
- If you have a strong fitness identity, you are far more likely to exercise consistently. And by exercising more often, you can build a stronger fitness identity - the more you exercise, and the more it becomes part of your daily life, the stronger your exercise identity will become, further reinforcing your desire to exercise and enjoyment from doing so.
- So habits - or the right ones - are fundamental to developing your exercise identity. The goal ceases to be to exercise, or to get thinner, but instead it is to become an exerciser, because that is the person you believe yourself to be.
- By making small, incremental changes on a daily basis, we can reinforce the behaviours of the person we wish to be.

- The results will come - they are the side effect of creating the right habits. And those habits will help you see yourself as the person you want to be, so that doing the things that person does will become second nature.

NEXT STEPS

Thinking of your destination goal, answer the following questions in your journal to gain a deeper understanding of who you need to become and how you can start acting now, to achieve your goals.

1. Who do you need to be to achieve this goal?
2. What is your "I am..." statement? For example, *"I am a runner"* (rather than *"I go running sometimes"*). Or *"I am an exerciser"*, or *"I am calm and have time to prioritise my fitness"*.
3. Describe the ideal day of this version of you.
4. What do you do?
5. What do you wear?
6. How do you think, act, interact?
7. What do you notice is different about this version of you?
8. What will you start doing NOW to bring the future you into reality? Hint: use your process goals.

10

BECOME THE ARCHITECT OF YOUR BEHAVIOUR

Our focus on getting motivated to exercise can often cause us to overlook one of the most important influences on our ability to exercise - our environment. The things that surround us on a daily basis, like people, objects, colours, sounds, smells, buildings and so on, are crucial contributing factors that drive our habits and behaviours. Your environment is one of the most powerful, invisible forces that shapes your life and it's far more productive to direct your energy into optimising your environment than trying to locate your lost willpower. No matter what your goal is, making small changes to your surroundings and the people you spend time with can have a profound effect on achieving a successful outcome and maintaining it. In this chapter, we will look at your physical environment and in the next chapter, your social environment.

Losing weight, building muscle, and improving stamina is incredibly difficult when your environment is working against you. You don't want to have to fight an uphill battle every day just to make small steps forward. If you want to live a longer and healthier life (with a toned, strong body that will naturally come with that), changing aspects of your physical environment is key.

THE BLUE ZONES

The most interesting example of the importance of your environment for longevity is the research conducted on the so-called "Blue Zones". Blue zones are regions of the world thought to have a higher than usual number of people who live much longer than average (for more than 100 years) without health issues like obesity, cancer and heart disease. The five blue zones identified by the longevity expert and National Geographic Fellow, Dan Buettner, alongside Gianni Pes and Michel Poulain are: Sardinia, Italy; the islands of Okinawa, Japan; Nicoya Peninsula in Costa Rica; Ikaria, Greece; and Loma Linda, California.

The team of researchers put together their findings to uncover the common habits and secrets of the healthier, happiest, and longest living people on earth. What they discovered was that their physical environment is perfectly designed to make healthy decision-making easier and, in some cases, completely mindless. Here are some examples of how their environment has shaped their healthy habits and behaviours: *Landscape -* none of these people took part in *voluntary physical exercise* as we understand it - running on a treadmill or going to the gym. This is because they have to walk almost everywhere. For example, in Ikaria in Greece, where the landscape is generally hilly and mountainous, a short walk is already a workout in itself. These people also have to grow their own food and so they often spend a large proportion of their time outdoors gardening and are involved in some form of manual labour. Regular exercise is a by-product of the design of their environment.

Home design - in Okinawa, most of their rooms don't have easy access to chairs, so they would naturally have to sit down on the floor. When they start to feel uncomfortable, they get up and move around. This means they get up to walk around up to 30 times a day. They don't need to be reminded by an app to do this. Likewise, the Sardinians live in vertical houses, so they have to continuously climb up and down the staircases to move around. Okinawans live seven years more than the average American, with one fifth the rate of cancer and cardiovascular disease.

Architecture - these people typically interact with each other on a daily basis. They have a tight knit community of support and this is due to the close proximity of each building and infrastructure. This close community contributes to the general happiness of the population because they are rarely isolated and everybody has a purpose in the larger community, including older people, who are respected and celebrated for their wisdom.

Objects - the Okinawans eat from a much smaller plate than our bigger western designs. Without even thinking about it, this strategy prevents overeating and piling on the calories. They also have very little access to devices like mobile phones, laptops, tablets and other technology that would distract them from being productive, or disrupt their quality of sleep. *Community* - these close communities take 24 hours once a week to completely shut down their work, spend time with family and visit their local faith-based institutions. Do you remember when that was a thing on Sundays, back in the day? This helps them to de-stress and unwind from a long week of hard work (manual work, remember!). They share similar interests, habits, and healthy lifestyle choices, which makes it much easier to maintain when everyone else is doing the same. I know some of these landscapes, designs and strategies are not practically possible to replicate in our current day lives. We are not all about to move to Okinawa to achieve longevity and nor should we need to. And you may not even be interested in living to 100! But if you want to live a comfortable life, free from aches and pains, with full mobility and body confidence by being consistent with your exercise, we have a lot to learn from these communities. And we can do this by looking at how to reverse engineer the Blue Zone design strategies and apply them in our everyday lives to get us moving more.

POWER 9

The group of medical researchers, anthropologists, demographers, and epidemiologists distilled their findings from the

Blue Zones into nine common denominators, or longevity lessons, which they called "Power 9". These are:

1. **Move naturally** throughout the day
2. Have and cultivate a strong sense of **purpose**
3. **Downshift** every day to relieve stress
4. **80% Rule:** stop eating when you are 80 percent full
5. **Plant Slant:** Make beans, whole grains, veggies, and fruit the centre of your diet
6. **Wine @ 5:** Enjoy wine and alcohol moderately with friends and/or food
7. **Belong:** Be part of a faith-based community, or organisation
8. **Loved Ones First:** Have strong family connections
9. **Right Tribe:** Cultivate close friends and strong social networks

It is the first of these lessons that we are most interested in, though finding your unique reason to exercise (sense of purpose) and relieving stress (downshifting) are also crucial when it comes to your motivation and succeeding in achieving your fitness goals. We will discuss lessons 7-9 in the next chapter on your social environment.

YOUR PHYSICAL ENVIRONMENT AND THE IMPACT ON YOUR BEHAVIOUR

In the modern western world, we look for the most convenient way to do things. We are programmed to choose the path of least resistance. We design our houses with convenience in mind, so we can throw laundry down a chute direct to the utility room, we have robotic vacuum cleaners and remote control mops, we can order healthy pre-prepared meals to our door and shop online for pretty much anything we desire (and often don't need). We have boiling water taps, instant ice dispensers, robotic lawn mowers, internet enabled ovens for remote cooking and even self-driving cars are on their way. Technology means we can even work on the sofa at home, in our pyjamas.

We are moving less because we don't need to. We can be completely sedentary and the world keeps turning. We have allowed ourselves to become physically passive in our own lives. So much so, that we don't even notice how we are influenced all day long by environmental factors. For example, when we walk into a quiet space, like a library, we automatically whisper.

With our environment shaping our behaviour, our habits are dependent on us optimising our surroundings. So how do we spend more time moving naturally throughout our day?

HOW TO DESIGN YOUR ENVIRONMENT TO MAKE EXERCISE HAPPEN

Every habit is initiated by a cue, or trigger and we use environmental cues all the time. The traffic light turns red, we use the brake to stop the car. We get something sticky on our hands, we wash them. The doorbell rings and someone in the family goes to answer the front door.

We are more likely to notice these cues if they stand out in our environment. For example, remembering to take supplements is something I have worked on for years. I keep them in a cupboard because I like tidy and uncluttered kitchen surfaces (though I rarely manage to achieve this). Because I can't see the supplements, I constantly forget to take them. So I moved them to a cupboard that was near the fruit bowl in the hope this would prompt me to take them. Still, I forgot to take them. The only way I can manage to take these daily supplements is if I have them out on the kitchen surface next to the cutlery drawer where I reach for a spoon every morning. It's not easy to remember to take them if they are hidden away in a cupboard.

Likewise, exercise is not top of mind when our mat is put away out of sight, and is not convenient when the gym is a 15 minute drive in the opposite direction to the office. It's not easy to remember to drink enough water if we never feel thirsty and don't have a bottle of water in front of us all day.

Your visual and auditory cues

Your habits depend on what you *see* and what appears to be convenient. The human body has about 11 million sensory receptors and approximately 10 million of these are dedicated to sight. To form and maintain good habits therefore, you must ensure that the right visual cues exist in your environment. You need to see something that flips a switch in your head to "go" and begin your workout.

If you are fairly new to exercise, visual cues in your environment will be key for you in getting started and creating this new habit. Once the habit has formed, the visual cues become less important.

The good news is, you can become the architect of your behaviour when you design your environment to support obvious visual (and to a lesser degree auditory) cues.

EXAMPLES OF HOW TO DESIGN YOUR ENVIRONMENT

- If you want to exercise first thing in the morning, put out your workout clothes near your bed the night before.
- If you want to get to your exercise class on time, set an alarm.
- If you want to remind yourself to get up from your desk to stretch after you've sat for a set period of time, set a timer.
- If you want to drink more water, fill water bottles and place them in the rooms you will be spending time in, or in your car to travel with you.
- If you want to spend more time reading on the sofa instead of watching mind-numbing reality shows, place your book on the sofa ready for when you arrive home.
- If you want to eat more fruit, place the fruit in a bowl that you have to walk past every day in the kitchen.
- If you want to do 5 press ups every time you use the bathroom (at home of course!), post a note on your bathroom mirror to remind you after you wash your hands.

As you can see, these cues can start out being very specific. However, over time these habits become associated not just with a single trigger, but with the entire context surrounding the behaviour.

Understand the context

Heading to the gym before work, or to your local park on a Saturday morning for the Park Run, puts your exercise into context. At the gym there will be multiple cues for you to exercise: seeing the gym equipment, watching others workout, hearing the pumping music, meeting your personal trainer, or working out alongside a friend. We mentally assign our habits to the locations in which they occur. The location develops a connection with the habit, or routine, of exercise, so when you arrive at that location, you move your body.

It's easier to form a new habit in a new environment because you're not fighting old cues. If you have used your kitchen for the same habits for years (eating, socialising, cooking, drinking), you're going to have a fight on your hands when you try to incorporate a new habit of exercise in the same context.

Similarly, if you are exercising in your study (where you work), the same issue arises. And when contexts overlap like this, it's easier for the easiest action to win out. So, in the kitchen, you are more likely to reach for a snack than do your workout, or in the study, you are more likely to hop on your laptop because you just remembered you forgot to send that email.

If you are able to provide a dedicated room for exercise in your home, great! But this isn't always practical. But all is not lost. If you are not able to change environments, you can redefine, or rearrange yours to create different associations. And predictable environments make it easier to adopt a healthy exercise habit.

Make "zones"

If you are working from home, as many of us increasingly are, there may be some overlap in the use of rooms for different behaviours. You may be eating, exercising and helping with homework in the kitchen. Or eating on the sofa in front of the TV. This can lead to overlapping contexts, which we want to avoid when we are looking to create new healthy habits.

A great strategy to overcome this is to create zones for different behaviours, such as only eating at the table, or only working at your desk. If possible, create a separate room, space, or zone for exercise. If you don't have a separate area for exercise, create a zone in one room that has your mat laid down, all your exercise equipment (if you are using any) and a water bottle to ensure you are keeping hydrated. You can set up your tablet here if you are following online workouts. Keep it simple and try not to use this space for anything else, like eating, relaxing, or studying / working.

Over time, you will be able to create a relationship with this new area that you associate with exercise. If you exercise on your mat when you go into the lounge first thing in the morning, over time, walking into the lounge in the morning becomes the trigger for exercise, not the specific action of getting onto your mat. You are associating being in the lounge at that time of day with moving your body.

These contextual cues reduce the thinking process related to each step in the process and instead, roll them up into one "mega action" that triggers the behaviour automatically. "*After I wake up, I roll out of bed and into my workout gear and trainers, head out of the door, and go for my morning walk*".

Start thinking of your environment as filled with relationships rather than objects. Your unique relationship with objects, or areas of your home, is useful in training your brain to view a particular part of your environment in a particular context. But to create better habits, you need to ensure that each object, or space, is only associated with one context.

Get creative

This creation of new zones at home can also help you to avoid adopting and maintaining old habits you would like to change, such as a daily wine drinking habit, chocolate habit, late evening social media scrolling habit, or lack of exercise habit. This happens when your environment becomes predictable. If you find this is happening, then the easiest solution is to change your environment in some way to make these unwanted habits more inconvenient and reframe the idea of traditional exercise to make it more convenient.

Convenience often arises as an obstacle to regular exercise, including:

- It takes too much time to workout
- It's a pain to drive to the gym
- It takes too long packing up all the equipment each time
- The timing of the class doesn't work for me
- I keep forgetting things I need for my workout
- I'm not sure how to use any of the equipment, or which weights to use
- Taking a shower after my workout adds on too much time.

We are conditioned to see exercise as something that needs to take place for a set amount of time each day, but how about if the emphasis becomes on moving in a more varied way throughout your day?

Are you able to change your movement patterns at home? We focus so much on making things as convenient as possible, but how about making some of your daily habits a bit more inconvenient, in order to move your body more. For example, if you always place your dinner plates on the upper left hand corner of the bottom shelf in the cupboard, what happens if you move them to the upper right hand corner of the top shelf? Making changes to your environment in this way requires slightly different movement patterns than the ones you are used to.

Another strategy that works is to place exercise equipment somewhere it doesn't traditionally belong to make using it much more convenient. Following my ankle surgery in early 2022, I have had a balance board in my kitchen and a Bosu ball in my lounge. If I'm chatting with my family in the kitchen, or waiting for dinner to cook, I will hop on the balance board for a few minutes to improve my ankle strength and overall balance. If I'm in the lounge relaxing, or watching TV with my children, I will use the Bosu ball. I started out balancing on the ball for my ankle strength, but I now regularly flip it over and do a short abs workout.

At first, having these boards in the kitchen and lounge was quite novel, but as time has gone on, I have got used to the idea of moving in short spurts of time throughout the day and

I am doing it more and more frequently. An additional benefit is that I now find my children on the boards chatting to their friends and playing around and experimenting with what their body is capable of. Yes, it gets competitive, but they are moving without being told to and without seeing it as "exercise". This is exactly what the communities in the Blue Zones are doing.

And you can get as creative as you like (depending on how orderly you like your house to be, of course). We recently put up a pull-up bar in the doorway to the spare bedroom. This way, every time I walk past the room (which is next to my study), I will do some pull-ups. Varied movement has become part of my day because it's convenient. The equipment is not hidden away in the garage and there is no real effort in using it because it's right in front of me. Not only has the equipment become a visual cue to exercise, but the placement of them has made it all much more convenient.

It is a different type of movement habit that enhances whatever formal exercise routine I choose to do in my dedicated space at home. And this has a ripple effect. Lately, I have observed my daughter using our stairs banister as a barre to practice her ballet.

An opportunity for movement

Movement, no matter how small, creates more movement. If the goal is to alter behaviour and improve basic mobility and strength, making small changes to the environment in which we spend the most time will cause small changes in how we move and how we interact with our surroundings. These small changes can lead to bigger changes over time, until the familiar environment is no longer a place just for rest and relaxation; it becomes an opportunity for movement.

This has, of course, been one of the most powerful things to come out of the Covid pandemic. Our view of our home environments was forced to shift if we wanted to continue a regular movement routine. Many of us also had to alter our home space to cater for homeschooling our children, but we did it out of necessity. We all had to alter our behaviour to accommodate other family members who were now in our space. So you can see how, with the right input, habits can change, sometimes making a deep shift in the way we lead our lives.

YOUR TENDENCY AND THE ENVIRONMENT

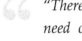
"There is a myth, sometimes widespread, that a person need only do inner work... that a man is entirely responsible for his own problems; and that to cure himself, he need only change himself... The fact is, a person is so formed by his surroundings, that his state of harmony depends entirely on his harmony with his surroundings." [1]

— CHRISTOPHER ALEXANDER

It's easier to change our surroundings than it is to change ourselves. Yes, there is inner work to do but whilst gaining a greater understanding of what makes us tick in order to get us moving more is the main thrust of this book, we shouldn't discount the power of our environment.

Take a good look at your environment to see if there are some simple changes you can make to support you in your efforts. Then we will move on to look at your social environment.

TENDENCY	PHYSICAL ENVIRONMENT	TAKEAWAY
Upholder	• Ensure you have a diary/calendar to record when you will exercise. • Monitor your progress with a tracker which is placed where you can see it each day.	Follow the plan.
Questioner	• Have the relevant information you need about an exercise regime to hand and know what you are doing and why. • Track your progress by wearing a device to track your steps or use an app to track when to hydrate or take your supplements, or chart what time you go to bed.	Focus on the data.
Obliger	• Monitor your exercise to support any accountability you receive. • Have your chosen method of accountability visible to you during the day - a workout calendar, app, commitment to attend a class with a friend, a challenge tracker etc.	Make your commitment visible.
Rebel	• Exercise as soon as you feel like it. Don't try to commit to scheduling exercise. • Make exercise convenient by getting creative with your environment so you can move when it suits you.	Create an environment where you can exercise your way whenever the mood strikes.

CHAPTER SUMMARY

- Your physical environment has a profound effect on how you live your life. Directing some energy into optimising your physical space, even in small ways, can have a big impact on behaviour and help to form new habits that support your goals.
- You can shape your preferred behaviours by designing your environment, like your home, to support positive visual and other cues.
- Create a separate designated space (a room or a zone in a room) for exercise, with your equipment, water bottles etc. ready and on hand.
- Over time, your relationship with this area will become associated with exercise.

NEXT STEPS

Draw your attention towards your environment and consider any changes you can make so it becomes more predictable for exercise. To do this, start by answering the following questions in the table below:

1. What parts of your environment currently support you in the achievement of your goal to exercise? What, if anything, makes it feel convenient?
2. What parts of your environment currently hinder you from achieving your goal to exercise? What, if anything, makes it feel inconvenient?

3. What will you change in your environment to make your goal of regular exercise a reality? To help you with this, think about:

- How you can scatter visual cues throughout your environment to remind you to move.
- Make a list of ways to incorporate movement into your day through changes in your environment. How can you make exercise more convenient?
- Think about assigning an area, or zone, at home for your workouts.
- Can you identify the problem that is stopping you from exercising? E.g. Is it really that you are not motivated to go for a walk early in the morning, or is it that you feel invisible, or unsafe, walking alone in the dark? In which case, buying a high vis vest to wear, or going with a friend might be the answer.

MY PHYSICAL ENVIRONMENT		
WHAT HELPS ME?	**WHAT HINDERS ME?**	**WHAT WILL I CHANGE?**

11

SURROUND YOURSELF WITH THE RIGHT PEOPLE

What is in close proximity to us, has an impact on us and shapes our habits and behaviours. This is true for our physical environment and also our social environment - the people we spend time with.

From childhood, we have an innate understanding of who our tribe is. We want to belong. Growing up, I was dedicated to my dance training, but it was made all the easier because I had a group of friends who had the same passion and were taking part in multiple classes a week. We practically lived at dance school. Added to that, my family all exercised on a regular basis. It wasn't just normal, it was enjoyable, and I had people to inspire, encourage, and support me.

We are social creatures and even our ancestors rarely exerted themselves alone. Hunter-gatherers foraged in groups, enjoying each other's company as they walked to find food. We have seen that the people living in the Blue Zones do the same, where resources can be scarce and communities have to help one another. We are programmed to assist each other in this way and we care what others think of us. So, when friends join a running club, or work out together at Cross Fit gyms, or play team sports, they are following on from the tradition of social physical activity. We cheer each other on when we succeed and encourage when we see someone struggling.

If you surround yourself with people who are fit and are moving on a regular basis, it is very hard not to do so yourself. Our close friends and family provide an invisible peer pressure that pulls us in the same direction.

POWER 9

We saw in Power 9, that three of the nine common denominators, or longevity lessons, distilled from the Blue Zones findings, are:

1. **Belong:** Be part of a faith-based community, or organisation
2. **Loved Ones First:** Have strong family connections
3. **Right Tribe:** Cultivate close friends and strong social networks

As we will see, these social connections are vital, not only in terms of motivating ourselves to exercise, but also when it comes to receiving support in doing so. In Okinowa, it is customary to form close bonds within local communities. A *moai* is an informal group of people with common interests who look out for one another. Serving the community in this way becomes their purpose. The moai originated when farmers would get together to share best practices during hard times and help each other with modest harvests.

Members of the moai make a set monthly contribution to the group, which allows them to participate in meetings, dinners, games or any other hobby they have in common. The funds collected are used for activities but if there is any surplus, one member (on a rotating basis) receives a set amount. This helps them to feel emotionally and financially stable. This feeling of belonging gives a sense of security and helps to increase life expectancy.

YOUR TRIBE

We can apply similar principles as the moai to assist with our desire to remain fit and healthy while living our modern life-style. For me, this would be to find a group of like-minded women in their mid-forties and beyond, who want to be fit and healthy into old age. When I have found my tribe, not only are they inspiring me to become a better person and sustain my healthy habits, but I am supporting them along the way, because I understand them, I know how they are feeling, the challenges they are facing in life and how sometimes, they just need someone to listen, rather than tell them ALL the things they should be doing right now. I also become someone who can tell them some home truths when necessary, rather than bark orders at them like a sergeant major. And they will do the same for me.

Developing a strong community bond like this means we prioritise our commitment to the group and we are constantly reminded of our healthy habits and why we have chosen them, and know exactly how to sustain them. It helps us feel stable in our efforts to meet our health and fitness goals, both emotionally and practically. On a practical level, our group can accompany us to the location where we are exercising, they can assist us with any information we may need and also participate alongside us. Emotionally, they can give us encouragement, welcome us to the group and give us a sense of belonging.

YOUR MENTORS

Another important piece of this jigsaw are the people who are supporting you professionally, whether that is your GP, a nutritional therapist, a personal trainer, a fitness professional leading your classes, a sports therapist, masseur / masseuse, or a physiotherapist. These individuals can be your guiding light, your mentor, advisor, and friend, supporting you in your efforts to achieve your goals. With their unique skills, they will be able to steer you in the right direction according to your individual physiology, age, existing health condition, and physical ability. They can monitor your progress, ensure your safety, provide discipline where needed and push you to your healthy limits. They can assist with use of equipment, give you feedback, and provide you with the crucial ingredient to success - self-awareness.

If I look at my journey with my health and fitness, I am very grateful to now have this team of professionals supporting me as I navigate the inevitable changes as I age. From doctors and nutritional therapists who have helped me through all the tests for perimenopause, to my physio following my accident and ankle surgery, and my sports therapist who helps keep my body free from aches and pains each month. I have learnt so much from these people, not only about the strategies we can deploy to optimise our health and fitness, but also about me and my body and how everything I am feeling and experiencing is normal. I now have a far better understanding of my body - what it needs and what it can struggle with. This is empowering and puts me in a much better position to future-proof my body. It also puts the brakes on any negative self-talk regarding my ability, or the changes I'm seeing in my body. Most importantly, it allows me to be kind to myself and show myself compassion when things are not going my way. Because they don't. On a fairly regular basis!

I would encourage you to take every opportunity to learn more about your body. If you are experiencing knee pain, don't ignore it. Go and find an expert who can help you understand what is going on. When you have the knowledge from one expert, you can find another expert to help you find different ways of moving, or adapting your current workouts. Never give up on yourself. There is always a way around injury, or a medical condition, and you can find the help you need. Don't take no for an answer when it comes to your physical wellbeing. Where there is a will, there's a way, so keep pressing to find the right support.

IMITATING HABITS

So how does our tribe help us? James Clear suggests that we tend to imitate the habits of three different groups:

1. The Close
2. The Many
3. The Powerful

The Close

We imitate those who are close to us. Our immediate family, partner and friends. We soak up the qualities of the people around us, so, as you can see, if you are living with a partner, or are hanging out with close friends who do not have the same health and fitness goals as you, and exhibit the behaviours that you are trying your best to change, this is going to be much harder for you.

On the flip side, if you are spending time with fit, healthy people, whose daily habits you are striving to imitate, you are more likely to consider these habits as normal behaviour, and in addition, see working out to be a common habit. Joining a culture where your desired behaviour is the norm is one of the most effective things you can do.

That said, joining a culture where you have little in common with the group is not necessarily going to help you. For example, if you join a running club and all the members are young 20-year-old men, you are unlikely to have much in common with them, even though your desired behaviour (running) is the norm in this group. Whilst hanging out with men half your age is appealing to some (!), you may feel out of place unless you have another common interest (e.g., you are all Schitt's Creek fans), and this means that change is less appealing to you because these people are not like you. You need to find a group of like-minded people, so you can see that the desired change is something that people like you are already doing. Your personal quest then becomes a shared one and there is nothing like belonging to a tribe to sustain your motivation to move.

The Many

We also imitate the behaviours of the many - the group. Whenever we are unsure how to act, we look to see what the group is doing. Have you ever walked into a crowded room in an unfamiliar setting and looked around to see what others are doing, in order to help guide your behaviour? We use reviews on Amazon and TripAdvisor and can be swayed by the number of people we are told have previously purchased an item to help us make decisions when we are buying a new product, or booking a holiday.

The reward for imitating the group is being accepted and we would rather have this than stand out from the crowd. We all want to conform (unless you are a Rebel of course!) and the reward of being accepted into a group can help you to change and maintain your habits. When changing your habits means fitting in with the crowd, change is very attractive.

The Powerful

Imitating the powerful is an interesting one that immediately got my back up. I'm not someone who strives to be powerful, or cares about status, but we are all drawn to behaviours that earn us respect, approval and admiration, even if we won't admit to it! This is why we are fascinated with successful people. We want to learn how they did it because we want success ourselves, whether that's in copying a recipe from our favourite baker, or using the same marketing tactics as someone successful in the online space, or taking up the latest fitness programme from a celebrity we follow and admire.

Other people have a huge influence over us. It is inspiring to be around individuals who are good role models. I have personally picked up lots of small habits by noticing what others are doing, or by hearing someone talk about something new they are doing. For example, I now "surf" on the London Underground trains rather than holding onto one of the hand rails, or sitting down. This was after I listened to a story on a podcast about a 79 year old man who was experimenting with moving in a more varied way each day by either surfing the Underground, or doing pull ups on the overhead handrails. I'm not quite brave enough to start doing pull ups on the train (my kids would also kill me), but no-one notices that I'm not holding onto anything.

I also try to do several press ups every time I use the bathroom (at home, not in public!) after learning about anchoring new habits to an existing habit (we looked at this in Chapter 7). My son is also a huge inspiration. He loves Parkour and rarely travels in a traditional way! He climbs onto things, hurls his body over objects and is constantly up a tree or lamp post (I once lost him on the walk home from school when I was busy chatting with a friend only to find him above my head up a lamp post).

THE DANGER OF THE WRONG TRIBE

Conversely, if our friendship group or close family circle are not exercising, we are unlikely to be doing so. A study in the United States, which tracked 12 thousand people for 32 years, found that if you have a friend who is obese, there's up to a 57% chance you'll become obese too.[1] Among pairs of adult siblings, if one sibling became obese, the chance that the other would become obese increased by 40%. If one spouse became obese, the likelihood that the other spouse would become obese increased by 37%. We want to belong to a tribe and if that tribe is overweight, we will follow suit.

SHIFTING YOUR SOCIAL ENVIRONMENT

So, what can you do to improve your social environment without waving goodbye to all your friends and family? Being with a group of like-minded women, who have similar health and fitness goals, helps to shape and reinforce your personal identity. This could be at a running club, in a sports team, at your local yoga class, or inside an online membership. The friendships you will make inside this new community will help to embed a new identity to sustain your motivation to exercise.

When it comes to your friends and family and the support they provide, Rubin describes them as falling into three "gears".[2] You may recognise one of these gears in a partner, or friend, who has tried to support you before. Or you may see yourself here if you have actively supported someone in reaching their goals.

People in "**drive**" mode add energy and force to habits. They can be helpful and encouraging and sometimes join in. But if they are too pushy, they could become irritating and cause opposition, especially with a Rebel. People in "**reverse**" try to reverse you out of a healthy habit. This can be from a sense of love, "*You should just let your hair down and enjoy yourself*", or the behaviour may be mean spirited, as they try to discourage you from sticking to a healthy habit (more often because of their own jealousy or guilt at not adopting the healthy habit themselves). Others are "**neutral**" and go along with our habits and support us in whatever we choose to do. This can be useful, but it can also be counterproductive because they just want us to be happy and this support makes it easier for us to indulge in some of our old habits.

Manage expectations

You don't have to ditch your friends (well, maybe not all of them) and start again. But you can be more mindful of creating healthy boundaries with friends who are not currently living a life that is in alignment with your values. You can manage their expectations by explaining that you will be spending some time focusing on your health and wellness over the coming months, which may mean you are spending less time meeting up for a glass of wine in the evening, or for coffee and cake at the weekend, and more time walking and completing your selected workouts. Either that friend will find something else to do while you are busy prioritising your health and fitness, or you will inspire them to join you on the journey.

Dealing with the naysayers

You may experience people around you actively undermining your efforts to change. Your new habit might be making them feel abandoned, or jealous of the healthy habit and its outcome, or guilty in the face of your efforts, or hurt if the habit makes them feel rejected, or judged. Or maybe they become annoyed because they see your new habit as a minor inconvenience to them, for example, if you have decided to workout in the morning and are no longer there to make everyone's breakfast. But if you make this habit a consistent one, they are soon going to have to get used to making their own breakfast. If it's an on-off habit, people don't have time to get used to it and may start to take it personally when you decide to go off and do your own thing.

Being able to recognise what you need, and who in your tribe is best able to help support you according to their "gear", is an important step in customising your social environment.

YOUR TENDENCY AND YOUR SOCIAL ENVIRONMENT

The table below highlights how your Tendency dictates what you need from your social environment. Social environment is key for Obligers.

TENDENCY	SOCIAL ENVIRONMENT	TAKEAWAY
Upholder	• Have a system of self-accountability - public announcement of your new exercise habit won't make much difference to you. • Spend time with fit, healthy people, whose daily habits you are striving to imitate. • You are unlikely to ask for support because you don't like to place the burden on others.	You are your best support.
Questioner	• Focus on your personal reasons for exercising, not on what others are doing. • Join a culture where your desired behaviour is the norm. • Know what results you can expect from a particular exercise regime - this is far more persuasive to you than any accountability.	Know which exercise regime you are doing and why.
Obliger	• Your social environment is critical to your success. • You must choose the right kind of accountability when it comes to exercise - in-person accountability from a trainer, coach, family member or friend. - a structured accountability group. - virtual support feels less intense if you are introverted. - face-to-face support if you enjoy being with others. • You could also think of yourself or your health condition in the third person (see below).	Systems of outer accountability are key to your success but choose which accountability works best for you.

Rebel	• You don't like being told what to do so you need to reframe situations. If you choose to use a personal trainer, instead of thinking *"This person expects me to do this exercise"* - which can trigger opposition - think, *"This person is doing what I want him to do so that I can get the result I want"*. • Tell yourself *"I can do whatever I want, and I want to exercise"*. • You can benefit from spending time with those whose habits you are striving to imitate and may also benefit from joining a group of like-minded women to support your efforts.	You are in charge, so reframe your thinking if necessary when receiving help from others.

One interesting method of creating outer accountability that sometimes works for Obligers is to think of themselves, or their health condition / injury in the third person: *"I hate going to the gym, but future me will wish I'd stuck to my workout schedule even though current me hates it"*. This is something that worked for Sheila, 67, who was diagnosed with type 2 diabetes and was prescribed medication. She wasn't overweight, but associated diabetes with being overweight, so this didn't sit well with her identity as someone who had done yoga and Pilates for many years.

I received an email one day from Sheila asking me if I thought she would be able to cope with my ballet fitness classes. Sheila was concerned, primarily because of her age, but also because she hadn't previously done anything more strenuous than yoga and Pilates. She came to class and this then gave her the confidence to add in more online classes during the lockdown period. When she had her annual diabetic check up, the nurse wanted to know what she had been doing differently from the previous year. When Sheila explained she had been exercising regularly she was told to keep it up as her blood/sugar levels had come down and the medication alone wouldn't have achieved this. In the space of six months, Sheila had also lost almost half a stone in weight and 3cms off her waist as a by-product of exercising. She saw exercise as an obligation to her diabetes. This was the way she framed it that made the most sense to her.

The Obliger people pleaser can also reframe exercise as a benefit to others rather than of personal value. Equally, if they can tie their duty to being a good role model (doing it for their kids), they can more easily meet expectations.

This spillover benefit to others is particularly important when it comes to motivating an Obliger to exercise. Health tends to be an area where other people nag or admonish (or at least that's how it can feel sometimes). A doctor might tell an Obliger to lose weight or make certain lifestyle changes to improve their health. The expectation to exercise can feel externally imposed, but the impact on health falls wholly on the Obliger's shoulders. And this is where Obligers need to be careful because if the burden of outer accountability becomes too heavy, they may show Obliger rebellion. If they meet an expectation over and over again, they may then suddenly stop and refuse to meet that expectation anymore.

EXCUSES

Because Obligers act when they are held externally account-able, they can look for reasons to excuse themselves from that accountability. These excuses might be:

- I have been really good all day, so it's fine if I skip my workout.
- I will do it tomorrow.
- I haven't been exercising because I'm too busy running around after everyone else.
- I only have 15 minutes, so it's not worth it.
- This slice of cake doesn't count.
- I've already showered so I can't workout now.
- It will be neglectful to my children if I go for a run now.

Sometimes Obligers can rebel against all efforts to fine-tune their bodies with an excuse that can be disguised as an embrace of life, or an acceptance of who they are, so that the failure to pursue an exercise habit seems life-affirming - almost spiritual. I have seen this happen with some women who are overweight and championing the body positivity movement. *"I want to embrace myself, just as I am"*. And I agree, we should love our bodies, but not to the detriment of our health. If carrying excess weight is damaging for our health, and if our health is a priority, then we must be honest with ourselves and take action to create habits that will help us achieve our health and weight loss goals. For most of us, the real aim isn't to enjoy a few pleasures right now, but to build habits that will make us happy over the long term. Sometimes, that means giving up something in the present, or demanding more from ourselves.

Obligers struggle most often against the temptation of excuses, but if you are an Obliger and you are aware it is happening, you can put a stop to it.

Rebels don't make excuses to justify doing what they want to do. Upholders and Questioners feel a greater pressure from their own inner expectations that helps them to resist excuses. But of course none of us are immune!

WORKING OUT ALONE

What about exercising on your own, rather than in a group? Despite all the evidence above that demonstrates exercising in a social setting can be beneficial in terms of your motivation and enjoyment, it can also be enjoyable when done on our own. In some situations it can even be therapeutic and meditative when we get into that state of flow. It's certainly my preference because I am able to focus entirely on my own body and not become distracted by others. I think it's also because I spend a proportion of my time teaching ballet-inspired workouts and other movement forms to groups of women, so exercising on my own feels like time out just for me. But we are all different and it really doesn't matter how you are doing it, provided what you are doing suits you and your Tendency.

Some people prefer to find numerous ways of distracting themselves while working out by themselves - by listening to podcasts, or watching TV on the treadmill, for example - but for most of us, exercise is emotionally rewarding, which is why we tend to belong to clubs, gyms, sports teams, or virtual communities. However you choose to do it, if it's working for you, keep doing it!

CHAPTER SUMMARY

- We are all influenced in our behaviours by those around us - those close to us, those who are successful and who we respect, as well as society in general.
- If you surround yourself with people who are fit and move regularly, you are more likely to do so too. They will motivate you to move and support you in doing so.
- Find your tribe - like-minded women with whom you have things in common and who want to be fitter and healthy.
- Get help and support from experts (medical, nutritional, fitness etc.) as and when you need it, who can advise you on how to meet your goals.
- Recognise those in your social circle who can help or harm you achieving your goals and manage those relationships.
- We are all different - it doesn't really matter how you do it, provided what you're doing suits you and your Tendency.

NEXT STEPS:

1. ME SHEETS

I want you to start focusing on putting yourself at the centre of your day and prioritising what's important to you. Our needs can so easily slip to the bottom of the pile and when this happens, we are not always aware of how we are feeling, or what it is that we need. When we get ourselves organised in this way, we can start to see where we need support.

Create a "Me Sheet" like the one below. This is like a to-do list, but slightly different because you are actually going to feature on this one! There are three columns and you are firmly placed in the centre column. You can use the columns either side to separate out your other tasks, which might be work, or home admin, or children. My sheet has work on one side and everything else on the other side.

When you next come to prepare your to-do list for the week, use this sheet. Your challenge is to ensure you have something listed in the middle column at all times that is to nurture and nourish you. Some ideas are listed below:

IDEAS OF WAYS TO NURTURE AND NOURISH MYSELF

- Buy myself some flowers
- Complete my workouts
- Go for a walk with Lydia
- Finish reading my book
- Organise dinner with friends
- Spend 15 minutes a day alone doing nothing! (I call this the "Boredom Break". You are not allowed to do anything but sit still. Try it and see what comes up for you.)
- Ask for help with childcare on Wednesday

Here is an example of a Me Sheet you can use:

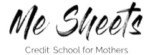

Credit: School for Mothers

ME

You can refresh this list every week but please make sure you have something in that middle column!

2. A LOOK AT MY SOCIAL ENVIRONMENT

This exercise is not intended to be a negative process. It's about bringing your awareness to the parts of your environment that are currently working for you and the gaps that may need filling in. You can use the table below, or use a spider diagram or map.

1. Looking at your three process goals from Chapter 7, start writing down ways in which your social environment may currently hinder your progress towards achieving these goals. This may or may not relate to particular people in your environment and it could be that you currently don't have the right accountability in place.
2. Next, write down ways in which your social environment could help you to achieve your goals AND any additional support / accountability / changes you may need.

MY GOAL	WAYS MY SOCIAL ENVIRONMENT HINDERS MY PROGRESS	WAYS MY SOCIAL ENVIRONMENT HELPS MY PROGRESS, OR CHANGES I CAN MAKE NOW TO HELP ACHIEVE MY GOALS
1.		
2.		
3.		

BODY AWARENESS

We are constantly faced with a barrage of information in relation to our health. Eat this, don't eat that, workout in the morning, it's better to workout in the evening, make sure you are following this exercise programme, workout for 5 days a week, and fast for 14 hours a day... It's all very confusing and unhelpful. But there is no workout that is going to work wonders for a 20-year-old male at the same time as reaping rewards for a 45-year-old woman.

Not everyone has the same body type, metabolism, dietary needs, or health limitations. Not everyone has the budget for a gym membership, or the confidence to take part in a fitness class. No one can walk our journey in life and they certainly don't get to tell us where it starts and where it stops. Only you can make decisions for yourself and take responsibility for your own body - a body that may benefit from losing a few pounds, or increasing muscle mass, or improving flexibility, or strengthening to improve your confidence, or simply moving to feel good. Our goals are different, our lives are varied and our physiology is unique to us.

Even within the four tendencies framework, there is variation in our mindset, behaviour, general outlook on life and ability to form habits. Up to this point in our lives, we have led a unique path with diverse experiences that have impacted the way we now process the world around us. If we can begin to understand our differences, what makes us tick, and become more self-aware of our changing female bodies, we are better placed to find the right strategies to optimise our health and fitness.

As a woman in my forties, I totally get the challenges that busy women in my age group face. Like it or not, despite our best efforts at exercising regularly and eating healthily, our bodies will change with age.

First, let's take a look and understand what is happening.

WHAT'S HAPPENING TO ME?

Did you know that in England, women are more likely than men to have a mental health problem and are twice as likely to be diagnosed with anxiety disorders?[1]

We are busier than ever

Dr. Libby Weaver goes some way to explaining why this might be. Rushing Woman's Syndrome (her 2017 book)[2] describes;

"the biochemical effects of always being in a hurry and the health consequences that urgency elicits. It's not a medical diagnosis but a title that reflects the changes happening in women's lives today".

There are many physiological impacts of being in this heightened state of rush (on your nervous system, endocrine system, hormones and bowels) and there are obvious mental health consequences too. Here are just a handful of the characteristics Weaver lists as typical for someone with Rushing Woman's Syndrome:

- Often feels overwhelmed;
- Can't sit down as feels guilty unless she is beyond tired;
- Answers 'so busy' or 'stressed' when asked how she is;
- Tends to crave sugar;
- Has a to-do list that is never completed; and
- Finds it difficult to relax without alcohol (which leads to increased body fat, cellulite, less energy and mood fluctuations).

Can you relate to any of these characteristics?

Obviously, not all mental health issues derive from being 'busy', but in my experience, so many women fall into this category. We are busy because we are at a time in our lives where we may be dealing with teenage children, taking care of elderly parents, working full time in a senior and responsible role, handling house admin, or supporting a friend going through a divorce or serious illness. Add into that a pandemic and perimenopause, we are being pulled in so many directions our heads are spinning. We have said "yes" too many times and there is now an expectation placed upon us to be there come rain or shine, at whatever hour of the day, for as many people who may need us. And we are good at it!

We cope. Just about.

It's only when we start to peel back the layers to understand why we don't ever seem to have time to workout, or frankly do anything we want to do just for us, that we start to see the problem. We are the problem. We have got stuck in a pattern of people-pleasing, or working ourselves into the ground in our career/business in order to feel like we are "good enough". Yes, we can blame it on others - our parents for messing us up, our children for being obnoxious, our partner for lacking empathy and not pulling their weight around the house - but these people are not going to suddenly change. By placing the blame outside of us, we are deferring responsibility to others, over whom we have no control. We are placing our health and happiness in their hands.

We have to take responsibility. We need to slow down. Specifically, we need to pay more attention to how our body feels, how it is changing as we age, so we can take back control and give it what it needs to feel great again.

We hit perimenopause / menopause

At the same time as our lives are becoming increasingly hectic, we hit perimenopause. Perimenopause is a transitional time that ends in menopause. Menopause means your periods have ended. When you have no menstrual cycle for a full 12 months, you have officially reached menopause. The average age for menopause is 51. Perimenopause can begin in some women in their 30s, but most often it starts in women aged 40 to 44. During perimenopause (which can last for 10 years or more), our levels of key hormones (oestrogen, progesterone and testosterone) start to decline. At the same time, we feel like our metabolism is slowing, our energy drops and we start to feel aches and pains in our body that weren't there before. It also takes us longer to recover from illness or injury. We notice that we are gaining belly fat and losing muscle mass.

Through the perimenopausal years, we can experience some, or many, of the following symptoms:

- hot flushes
- difficulty sleeping, which may be a result of night sweats
- palpitations, when your heartbeats suddenly become more noticeable
- headaches and migraines that are worse than usual
- muscle aches and joint pains
- changed body shape and weight gain, usually around the mid-section
- skin changes including dry and itchy skin
- reduced sex drive

- vaginal dryness and pain, itching or discomfort during sex
- recurrent urinary tract infections (UTIs).

We gain a few pounds

At this stage our bodies can no longer tolerate junk food, sugar and alcohol. Forget what we ate and drank in our 20s. That was then and this is now. We simply can't put away what we used to and "get away with it". This is a frustrating time as it means having to change our eating habits, particularly if we are no longer exercising as much as we once did.

In addition, if you have had babies, or lost a lot of weight, there will also be laxity in your muscles. They have been stretched and have lost their elasticity, which leads to the 'overhang' or 'apron'.

And it's not just about eating healthily and exercising regularly. You also need to consider your quantity and quality of sleep and your stress levels. These play a huge factor in gaining, or retaining weight.

We move less

We are also less active due to career and family demands. Long hours sitting at a desk, coupled with juggling the demands of family, mean we struggle to find the time to do ANYTHING for ourselves, let alone exercise. And if we don't particularly enjoy exercising, this is not going to be a priority when we get those precious free hours (minutes!) to ourselves. But we know we need to move for optimal health.

We experience increased levels of stress

We can start to experience a feeling of loss of control over our lifestyle because of the demands placed upon us. We might drink more to escape this reality and to take the edge off a busy day, or eat unhealthy foods as a "reward" for getting through it. In desperation, we also try fad diets and crazy bootcamps (which are, by definition, short-term and extreme) in a concerted effort to turn things around, but we are not consistent and so don't see the results we want.

Stress can have an impact on us physically and emotionally. When we are going through these times of stress, it's important to be aware of the impact that it's having on us, because the more knowledge we have about these things, the more we're inclined to try and do something about it, and to make positive steps to change things.

A study in 2018 by the Mental Health Foundation reported that 74% of people were overwhelmed, or felt unable to cope with daily life due to stress. 81% of women described themselves as stressed, compared to 67% of men.

There are some situations where your stress may be short lived, but there are so many other situations where your stress stays at a high level for a more prolonged period of time: the loss of a loved one, the loss of a job, an argument with your spouse, financial debt, health issues, comparing yourself to other people. All of these things can have a longer lasting effect on our physical and emotional well-being.

When we get stressed, our body releases a hormone called cortisol. This is the hormone that triggers the "fight or flight" response. The reason we have this is in case of an emergency. We are told by our body to either run away, or stay and fight. However, if we are in a situation where that stress response is being called on several times a day, day after day after day, that has an adverse effect on our body and can cause a number of different issues.

Stress can cause our breath to quicken, so we start to shallow breathe, which then makes us even more stressed. Our heart rate will start to quicken as well. Muscles become tense because you're ready for action (this is part of the fight response in the body that is preparing to save you in an emergency). You might experience headaches or migraines; you might get tension in the neck or shoulders because the muscles are so tight.

Another response from the body when we get stressed is to release acid in the stomach, which can lead to heartburn, which then has an effect on our digestive systems. It can cause insomnia, and then you become more stressed due to lack of sleep. It's a snowball effect.

Stress can also weaken the immune system, which means you are more prone to getting infections and viruses like the common cold. Aside from the physical and emotional effects of stress, it can also lead to cravings for things like sugar, salt, and carbs. In addition to that, when cortisol levels are high, the body actually retains weight.

When we are stressed, we are far less likely to carve out the time to move our bodies because it just feels like another chore on our never-ending to-do list at a time when we already feel exhausted. If we can slow down and reduce our stress levels, we can start to see the wood for the trees and begin to prioritise ourselves in order to counteract many of the side effects of stress. When we start exercising again, this in turn helps to reduce our stress levels and actually gives us more energy, as well as releasing hormones that improve the mood.

We feel the pressure

At the same time all this is going on, we are bombarded by social media images. Images of young and not-so-young celebrities looking beautifully tanned and slim, seemingly without making any effort whatsoever and living a far more reckless life than we are. But there are no quick fixes. The promises of a bikini body in seven days, or dropping two dress sizes by following the new workout plan or juice detox, makes us think this is actually doable (which of course, it isn't, certainly not sustainably or safely) and that we are a failure for being unable to achieve this. We assume it is our fault that we have no willpower.

Our self-confidence is challenged. Bottom line, we don't feel sexy anymore. Our identity has been compromised. We see wrinkles appearing on our face and grey hairs sprouting from our heads. We try desperately to take action to prevent this from happening, but we still don't feel good inside. We don't identify with the person we were before we had children, or when we were younger, and we feel a little lost. Plus, the idea of walking into a new exercise class or the gym fills us with dread. The fear of making a total fool of ourselves is paralysing.

Learning how to manage our body image is crucial as our bodies undergo these age-related changes. It helps us to focus on what really matters - our health.

We can't turn back the clock

In an attempt to remain young and vibrant, many women take action to retain their youthful appearance, from colouring their hair to hide the grey, buying expensive creams that promise to rid their faces of wrinkles and their thighs of cellulite, or ramping up the makeup routine, as well as more extreme things, like Botox, dermal fillers and surgery. This can work on a superficial level, but it doesn't help us to address the physical and emotional changes that are a natural part of the ageing process. Whilst it may go some way in alleviating any anxiety you may have over the way you look to the outside world, it will not protect you from age-related diseases such as atherosclerosis and cardiovascular disease, cancer, arthritis, cataracts, osteoporosis, type 2 diabetes, hypertension and Alzheimer's disease. The incidence of all of these diseases increases exponentially with age and older women are more likely than men to have chronic, or ongoing, health conditions.

I'm not asking you to like this ageing process, but you can't stop it. What you CAN do is to take steps to improve your health and fitness to reduce your risk of getting debilitating or life-shortening conditions. You can't turn back the clock, but you CAN embrace this new chapter in your life and fine-tune what you have so you can FEEL good about yourself again. This starts with self-awareness. Learning as much as you can about your own unique body and mindset. You are then far better placed to make the necessary changes to ensure you live a long and healthy life and to feel proud of how you present yourself to the outside world.

WHAT CAN I DO ABOUT IT?

So, what is the secret to living a life you love? It doesn't require an entire overhaul of your life. It necessitates some small changes in the way you think and the actions you take on a daily basis. Yes, it will take some re-wiring and will at times be uncomfortable, but it's the times you feel discomfort that you know you are moving on to greater things. You are growing and progressing, which is what you are meant to do.

If you are feeling overwhelmed with life right now and unable to find a way forward into a happier, healthier, calmer place, you need to realise that you are not alone. Many women have talked to me about the frustrations they have - feeling trapped, isolated and overwhelmed by work, children, household chores, and supporting family and friends, leaving little time for catching up with friends and having fun. And leaving less time for arguably the most important of all your roles, which is looking after yourself.

We all know that if we are not happy and healthy, we do not perform any of the above responsibilities well (or at all), leaving us feeling guilty, drained and stressed. When we try to carve out some "me" time, it is often sabotaged by any number of unexpected occurrences - like poorly children, a work deadline, friends cancelling at the last minute, or your childcare arrangements falling through - so then we decide that there is no point even trying. At least until the next time…

1. CREATE CLEAR BOUNDARIES

It's a Catch 22 isn't it? If you could find some time to yourself, to exercise and 'switch off' for an hour or so a week, you would feel more in control, more invigorated and able to deal with what life throws at you on a daily basis. In an ideal world, we would all find one hour a day to dedicate to exercising.

Back in the real world, we are lucky to find one hour a week. So much happens in a 24 hour period that exercising always seems to come at the bottom of a long list of tasks. Time is limited and precious. Which is why it is so important to ensure we are making good use of the time we do have, and blocking out time to make our well-being a priority. If you currently can't carve out time to prepare a healthy meal, or fit in a 15 minute workout, but are spending hours a week volunteering at school, this imbalance is an immediate sign you have boundary issues.

Signs you need boundaries include:

- Feeling overwhelmed.
- Feeling resentful towards people for asking for your help.
- Avoiding phone calls and interactions with people who might ask for something.

- You make comments about helping people and getting nothing in return.
- You daydream about dropping everything and disappearing.
- You have no time for yourself.

A lack of understanding about boundaries is what breeds unhealthy habits. We need boundaries for ourselves and for others. There are different types of boundaries - physical, emotional, sexual, intellectual, and material - but I'm going to talk about time boundaries for the purposes of this book, as it's the area women seem to struggle with the most.

Women with time boundary issues tend to struggle with work-life balance, self-care (which includes exercise), and prioritising their needs. Time boundaries consist of how you manage your time, how you deal with favour requests, and how you structure your free time. If you don't have time for something you want to do, you don't have healthy boundaries in place.

The healthiest way to communicate your boundaries is to be assertive. Tell the person who is asking to meet with you, *"I work from 9-5pm every day, so I'm not available to chat during that time."* To honour your time boundaries before you say yes to a request, check your diary first to make sure you are not over-committing. Don't try to squeeze in another event or task, or you will feel upset with yourself. When you're busy, allow calls to go to voicemail and texts to go unread unless it's convenient for you to respond.

Embrace guilt

Whenever I talk to clients about boundaries, one of the things that comes up most often is guilt. Women tend to feel guilty if they are saying no to others and prioritising their own needs. For example, spending time exercising instead of playing with their children, going for a walk rather than tidying the house, meeting a friend for a drink instead of spending more time on a work project. I'm not going to tell you to stop feeling guilty because by this stage, it is simply part of the process. You are not going to implement boundaries without feeling some pangs of guilt.

This is primarily because since childhood, we have been programmed to experience guilt for wanting to implement our boundaries. You may have had a parent who forced you to hug your Auntie Joan when you really didn't want to, telling you afterwards *"well that was mean"* or *"that wasn't very nice"*. It's manipulative behaviour to tell a child they are mean for not complying with a request. All we are doing is teaching them to feel guilty for attempting to honour their own boundaries. So, try not to treat your feelings of guilt as an adult as something that has to hinder your progress. It's just a feeling. Don't focus on the emotion and instead stay strong with your intentions. Obligers have a particularly hard time with boundaries and need to set up systems that encourage them to say no and make time for themselves. They are susceptible to burnout because they tend to be the go-to people when others need help. This can lead to them feeling underappreciated and resentful, and possibly exploited. However, if they feel overwhelmed by external pressure, they rebel and simply refuse to meet an expectation. They quit exercising, tell themselves they are hopeless and avoid it for a period of time, before returning and repeating the same pattern at a later stage. This can often happen in the area of health because others are nagging them to lose weight or exercise. To help them avoid rebelling, they need to recognise this behaviour pattern and set up those boundaries.

So, it's time to step out of your own way, reprogramme your thought processes and create time to improve your sense of well-being. Your family will thank you for it. Let's call this your "happy sweat". And it begins with saying "no" to other people more often, and "yes" to yourself at every opportunity. Place a boundary around that daily 15 minute workout and protect it.

2. REDUCE STRESS

Control the controllables

When it comes to reducing our stress levels, I always like to focus on controlling the controllables. There are events that we are in control of that can cause us stress and there are events that are completely outside our control. If we pay attention and take the time to analyse what is causing our stress, we can learn to reduce the number of stressful events that are within our control and, for those that are outside our control, we can learn to become more resilient.

If you take a look at your daily routine, you may be able to identify occasions that are relatively minor, but have the potential to disrupt the flow of everyday life and add to overall levels of stress. Mundane hassles (like rushing to get your child to a class on time after leaving the house at the last minute, transactions with others in everyday life (like the friend who is always leaning on you for advice but never asks how you are), or other annoyances associated with routine. Once you have identified the stressful situations, you can begin to work on making changes to your routine to try and eliminate the stress.

For example, instead of rushing to get to work on time because you have tried to squeeze in yet another load of washing before you leave, plan your week so you are doing the laundry on set days. That means you are not doing it minutes before leaving the house. Or plan to get up 10 minutes earlier on that day so you have time to complete any tasks in the morning. Give yourself plenty of time to get your children to their activities, or yourself to your weekly yoga class. Work with your partner to share out household responsibilities so that they work better for you. If you are working from home, turn off your laptop at a set time, so you can enjoy downtime with your family. Remember, if you have clear boundaries in place, this becomes much easier.

For the other routine occasions that are outside our control, like someone jumping the queue in the supermarket, or being stuck in a traffic jam, we are able to adjust our response to them. We are not in control of what others do and we don't want to hand them control over our happiness and health.

Instead of cursing the person who jumped the queue (under your breath of course, if you are British), you could choose to:

(a) say nothing - maybe they are in a rush to return to a sick relative; (b) kindly point out that there is a queue - maybe he/she didn't realise; or (c) if they ignore, or respond to your polite request in an aggressive manner, get creative with how you choose to feel in response. I have used it as a learning opportunity for my children (on how not to behave, of course) and also as an exercise in empathy - generally, unpleasant people are not happy people. This takes time and I am most definitely still a work in progress, but this change in mindset has made a significant difference to my daily stress levels.

Breathe and meditate

When you experience stress, your breathing pattern changes. You are likely to be taking small, shallow breaths, using your shoulders rather than your diaphragm to move air in and out of your lungs. Shallow over-breathing, or hyperventilation, can prolong feelings of anxiety by making the physical symptoms of stress worse. Controlling your breathing can help to improve some of these symptoms.

When you are relaxed, you breathe through your nose in a slow, even and gentle way. Deliberately copying a relaxed breathing pattern calms the nervous system that controls the body's involuntary functions. Controlled breathing can cause physiological changes that include lowered blood pressure and heart rate and reduced levels of stress hormones in the blood.

Take deep breaths several times throughout the day, this can be done while you're travelling to work, or if you're stuck in a traffic jam, or it can be done first thing in the morning to start the day as you mean to go on. Take deep breaths in through the nose and out through the mouth to calm your mind. This will help you reduce your cortisol levels.

Another fantastic way of helping reduce stress is meditation, which also uses controlled breathing to calm the body and mind. This is not something I did until very recently. I remember my mother doing it when I was child, but I never really understood it. If you are not sure how to get started, you could try a meditation app like Headspace, or Calm. Inside my BBackstage membership, we have pre-recorded meditations and breathing tutorials to help our members. If you've got a busy mind like I have, you have to train your mind as much as you would train your body if you were trying a new workout.

Exercise

We are talking about reducing stress so we can counteract the effects of stress on our body and mind, which in turn frees up some headspace to start carving out time to exercise. And of course one of the best ways of relieving stress is to exercise! So again, it's a bit of a Catch 22 situation. We are too stressed to exercise, but don't like the fact we are retaining weight around our midsection and yet the very thing we need to do to reduce our stress levels is exercise.

There is stronger evidence than ever before that movement not only improves your mental health, it also protects it. When we exercise, we produce a cocktail of hormones, including endo-cannabinoids – all of which contribute to making us feel good. Endorphins are produced at a certain intensity of activity, but the mood-boosting effects of exercise are felt at a much lower level. According to Jack Raglin, a professor of kinesiology at the Indiana University's School of Public Health, a single "dose" of exercise can improve your mood for several hours. But not only are the benefits "immediate and perceivable": with a regular regimen, they can accrue over weeks. *"In other words, there is a long-term and continual improvement,"*[3] he says.

So go for a walk with a friend instead of having that glass of wine in the evening. The movement, the fresh air, and talking to your friend will really help.

3. SLEEP

Focus on tidying up your sleep habits. What's the best way you can get eight hours of sleep a night? Inevitably, that will mean going to bed earlier. When you're feeling tired and wanting to go to bed, that's your body's alarm. When it goes off, don't then go and load the dishwasher, or put a load of washing in the dryer, or do all the other things that we do before we go to bed. It can wait until the next day. Your sleep is so much more important. Sometimes it works, sometimes it doesn't, life is not perfect, but really try and get that sleep in.

Making exercise part of your regular routine can aid a better night's sleep, which boosts your mood. It improves the *quality* of your sleep, because it increases the amount of time you spend in the deep sleep phase, and increases the duration of your sleep because it expends energy and makes you feel tired and ready to rest. In addition, because exercise reduces stress and anxiety (which are common causes of sleepless nights), you have a better chance of falling asleep with ease and having a restful night.

4. FOCUS ON YOUR NUTRITION

You need to adjust your food intake to account for your loss of muscle mass if you are no longer exercising, but don't focus on lowering your calorie intake because this may slow your metabolism down, which can result in weight gain. Eat wholefoods and include protein in every meal to stabilise your blood sugar and control your appetite, as well as lowering your intake of starchy carbs and refined sugar.

5. EXERCISE SMARTER

Our bodies benefit from three forms of exercise - cardio workouts, body strengthening, and restorative workouts (like stretching, or a gentle yoga session).

Cardio workouts can help us lose weight, feel confident and raise our self-esteem. But you may be pleased to hear that long cardio sessions are not the secret to weight loss/toning when we are in our 40s. If you do too much, it overtaxes your body and increases your levels of the stress hormone cortisol, causing belly fat. Your goal should be to add muscle to your body using your own body weight. Ballet fitness workouts are fantastic for this and will help you to achieve a strong feminine physique.

Restorative workouts help to calm the system down. Conscious breathing is crucial to restore calm. It is key to making the shift in your chemistry, including reducing stress. Focusing on your breathing during a yoga class, a stretch class, or any other restorative workout, can help us to tap into our autonomic nervous system, which controls relaxation/sense of calm.

Hands down, the best exercise you can do is body weight training, to build muscle and prevent any loss of muscle mass. Muscle is the most metabolically active tissue in the body so the more muscle you lose, the slower your metabolic rate, which can contribute to weight gain.

Menstrual cycle

If you are still having periods, tracking your menstrual cycle can really help when it comes to your exercise regime. If you are no longer having a monthly period, it's still a good idea to track your energy levels to see if there is a pattern each month. Often, we put pressure on ourselves to push on through with cardio workouts when we are already feeling depleted. This is unwise, particularly at certain times of the month.

During the **menstrual phase** of your cycle (approximately days 1 - 6), your oestrogen and progesterone levels nose-dive. This leaves you feeling exhausted. This is not a good time to do heavy hitting cardio sessions that will deplete you. Instead, at this time choose to do restorative work like stretching, gentle yoga, tai chi movements, or simply meditate.

In the **follicular phase** (approximately days 7-11) your oestrogen starts to rise. This can leave you feeling refreshed and with more energy for strength training.

During the **ovulatory phase** (approximately days 12-19), shortly before ovulation, your oestrogen and progesterone levels start to rise. At this time you may start to feel competitive, energised, and have loads of energy to do all your work-outs. This would be the time to push yourself with cardio, or strength training.

During the final **luteal phase** (approximately days 20-28), your hormones will start to peak. This can leave you feeling lethargic as they slowly decline before you head back into the menstrual phase. At this stage, you need to listen carefully to your body and adjust your workouts over this eight-day period. Sleep can be disrupted during this phase and so, if you find yourself sleep deprived, you will need to be careful to avoid injury.

The mind - body connection

Exercise promotes a mind-body connection. Adding a mind-fulness element to your workouts means that you are not only improving your physical condition, but you are interrupting a flow of constant worry. It enables you to 'switch off' and reconnect with your body. Your focus is taken away from obsessive thoughts, feelings of panic, and overwhelm, and instead is targeted towards your balance, movement and breath.

We know that if you fix your fitness mindset (your thoughts, feelings, beliefs, and attitudes), this means you move more frequently and it can positively affect your biological function-ing. In other words, our minds can affect how healthy our bodies are! But have you heard how powerful the reverse of this is?

A revolutionary new understanding of the mind-body connection is revealing how our thoughts and emotions don't just happen inside our heads, but that the way we move has a profound influence on how our minds operate.[4] This opens up the possibility of using our bodies as tools to change the way we think and feel.

Did you know that:

- Different running speeds provide different mental benefits?
- People who are stronger in middle age have more grey matter and better memory a decade later?
- Dancing with others provides us with a state of closeness and understanding, as well as a desire to help others?
- Upright, expanded posture brings a more positive mental attitude?
- Stretching helps move the body's fluids along, allowing the immune system to give these liquids a regular clean-out and deal with inflammation as it arises?

Mind blown.

If there was ever a reason to exercise, this is it! For all those Questioners out there, you should by now have a long list of reasons for moving your body that you may have been unaware of before!

CHAPTER SUMMARY

- We all have different body types, nutritional needs and health limitations and we all have different lives, affecting our minds and bodies.
- Learning how to manage our body image is crucial as our bodies undergo age-related changes, and will help us to focus on our health.
- We can't turn back time, but we can take steps to improve our health and fitness to improve our chances of having long, active, illness-free lives.
- It's ok to feel overwhelmed with life, but small changes can make a big difference.
- Be assertive in creating and protecting boundaries to support your health and fitness. Accept you may feel guilt about it, but that's just a feeling and will pass.
- Reduce stress by controlling the controllables - moving things around in your diary to work better for you, postponing or cancelling non-urgent tasks, not taking on new responsibilities etc.
- Take time to breathe or meditate and especially to exercise. Exercise is incredibly powerful in improving health (of both the body and mind) and fitness when done right, in time with your body.
- Don't forget about sleep - go to bed earlier to ensure you get a good 7-8 hours a night.

NEXT STEPS

1. BOUNDARIES

Create a list of boundaries that you would like to implement. For example, *"spend 15 minutes a day exercising"*. Next to each one, identify actionable steps you need to take to help you uphold your boundary.

MY BOUNDARIES	MY ACTION STEPS

13

DISCOVERING HOW CAPABLE YOU REALLY ARE

We have talked about the mental side of fitness and the environmental factors you can change to help support your exercise goals, but another really important part is choosing the right exercise for you in terms of your preferences, your temperament, and your capability. This chapter will address this issue, along with how to use your mental tools to practice self-compassion when the going gets tough.

THE ABILITY CHAIN

What can we do to ensure that we are embracing exercise as a skill and then actually doing it? Because let's face it, that's the most important part.

B.J. Fogg[1] suggests we put motivation to one side and take a look at our ability in terms of what we find hard to do and what we find easy to do. When we can manipulate ability, our habits take hold much more quickly than when we are relying simply on motivation. When you look at the exercise regime that works best for you, ask yourself, *"What is making this behaviour hard to do?"* Fogg says your answer will involve at least one of five factors in what he calls the "Ability Factors":

1. Do you have enough **time** to do the behaviour?
2. Do you have enough **money** to do the behaviour?
3. Are you **physically capable** of doing the behaviour?
4. Does the behaviour require a lot of creative or **mental energy**?
5. Does the behaviour fit into your current **routine** or does it require you to make adjustments?

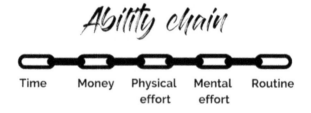

| Time | Money | Physical effort | Mental effort | Routine |

Is there a weak link somewhere in your Ability Chain? Which of the above factors is likely to cause you the most trouble? What is it exactly that stops you from exercising?

In order to make a habit easier, we need to identify what is making it feel hard right now. When you can identify which of these five links in the chain is or are causing your habit to feel difficult, you can focus on making it easier.

Let's look at an example. All my workouts inside my Breaking Ballet programmes are 10-15 minutes long. This sounds easy right? But the excuse I hear the most is lack of *time*. But we can burst through that belief fairly easily (as you have seen in Chapter 4). *Money* isn't necessarily an issue because they are doing the workouts from home and not paying for an expensive gym membership they never use. *Physical* effort most definitely makes the behaviour much harder as, even though the workouts are short, they are high intensity and take some grit to get through. So the *physical-effort* link could be weak here and that alone could be enough to derail your 15 minute workout habit. Then there is the *mental effort*, which we know can be a challenge. In addition, your *routine* may need some work, to get consistent with this new habit of exercise.

So, how do we make the habit of exercise easier? Specifically, in the above example, how do we make the physical and mental effort and our routine easier?

Fogg describes three approaches:

1. **Increase your skills** - with exercise, this takes practice and when you get better at your chosen form of exercise, it's easier to do. This requires you to do the same form of exercise over and over until you feel competent in it. If you are practising any of my ballet-inspired workouts, you may find an arabesque workout challenging for your balance, or a plié workout tough on your legs. But if you take the time to listen to the instructions about correct form and practice in short bursts on a consistent basis, your skill

will increase and the habit of exercise becomes easier.
The physical effort is reduced. (Of course, that's when
it's time to step it up as your biggest gains come when
you are pushing yourself).

2. **Get tools and resources** - you need to consider using
   some additional tools and resources as a catalyst for
   change. This could mean new walking / running
   shoes, a yoga mat to complete your workouts,
   comfortable workout gear that you enjoy wearing,
   establishing clear boundaries with family or friends,
   seeking accountability, or gaining access to online
   workouts that save you time and money. Difficulties
   with mental effort can be dealt with by preparing your
   schedule to remove decision-making and, by
   implementing a plan that sets a simple routine, your
   workouts will become more sustainable.

3. **Make the behaviour tiny** - regardless of your
   motivation levels, making your exercise habit as small
   as possible is a fantastic way to kickstart this daily
   habit and make it feel easier. If a 15 minute workout
   feels like too much at this stage, either because of a
   lack of fitness, or lack of time (but you know that's just
   an excuse right?!), reducing the exercise into a mini
   workout will get you started. Even if it's for two
   minutes. As explained in chapter 7, when it comes to
   creating a new habit of exercise, the length of time at
   this stage doesn't matter. It's all about holding space
   for the habit on a daily basis.

FITNESS IS A SKILL

Physical movements are skills. You may have been born with a natural aptitude for certain movements, but other movements may not feel as easy. If movement is not something you feel particularly confident with, you may need to consider what skills you need to develop. For example, if you have been told by a doctor to exercise for improved health, you need to change your behaviour. But you may have tried before and it was too challenging and became something you could easily avoid. If we look at your capability when it comes to movement, do you have the necessary skills to behave another way? If you have never had any guidance on fitness mindset, or how to move, what exercises to do and how often, it's not surprising that it feels challenging.

Like any skill, physical movement requires practice so we can hone our potential. Fitness success is not based on innate talent. If you are not currently exercising, this isn't the result of a flaw in character, lack of self-control, discipline, or intelligence. You need a mental map, a strategy and the requisite skills to achieve your goals.

Remember when you were a child learning to cycle or swim? How many times did you fall off that bike and graze your knees? How long did you wear armbands in the pool until you had the confidence to head into the deep end unaided? For the time you had stabilisers on your bike and wore armbands in the pool, you weren't telling yourself something was wrong with you, or that you lacked the discipline to learn these skills.

That's because you realised you just hadn't fully developed that skill yet. You would think about what was happening and be guided on how to progress, either by a parent, who ran holding the back of your bike once the stabilisers were off, or by the swimming instructor, who walked alongside the pool, encouraging you to keep kicking your legs. Success is reliant on improving your different skill sets through hard work, learning and experience.

However, when it comes to fitness, when we fail to complete a workout, or struggle to get ourselves co-ordinated in a class, we automatically beat ourselves up for being lazy, hopeless, and lacking in willpower. We don't take the time to think about why we have "failed". So when the same pattern happens next time we try to use willpower to force ourselves to complete the workout. What we need to do is figure out what is going wrong and apply a strategy that works for us.

If we can view fitness as a skill (rather than a talent), we can make a start on improving its component parts. This strips away any self-deprecating jokes and gives us something to work on. Breaking it down in this way helps us to see where we may be lacking the necessary skills, but also the areas in which we may already be excelling. Let's look at the three components of the fitness skill.

1. UNDERSTANDING THE OUTER GAME OF FITNESS

The "outer game" of fitness has to do with your physical skills (as opposed to your mental skills). For example, this might involve which types of exercises to do, how many repetitions to make, or when to exercise. The answers to these questions will, of course, differ for each individual. This knowledge allows us to create a plan and execute it.

Rubin identifies a number of factors that contribute to whether or not an exercise regime suits you.[2]

- Are you a morning person, or a night person?
- Do you enjoy being outdoors, or do you prefer not to deal with the weather?
- Are you motivated by competition?
- Do you enjoy exercising to strong music, and a driving beat, or do you prefer a quiet background?
- Do you respond well to some form of external accountability, or is internal accountability sufficient?
- Do you like to challenge yourself with exercise (learning a new skill, pushing yourself physically), or do you prefer familiar activities?
- Do you like sports?
- Is it inconvenient for you to take a shower after exercise?

Answering these questions will help you to decide whether a particular exercise regime is likely to suit you or not. Of course, exercise doesn't comprise a single skill and is made up of multiple skills that contribute towards optimum health:

Endurance - e.g. running or cycling at a moderate speed, or dancing

Stamina - alternating running with weight lifting

Strength - squatting (or doing some plies!), using resistance bands

Flexibility - stretching and mobility work

Power - Olympic lifts

Speed - sprint intervals

Co-ordination - dancing

Agility - Animal Flow, or box jumps

Balance - walking lunges, or an arabesque workout

Accuracy - the perfect serve in tennis

Looking at this list, and thinking about your fitness goals, is there a particular skill, or skills that you need to practice and improve on, in order to achieve fitness success? If your goal is to strengthen and tone your body, then the skills of strength, stamina, and agility might be high on your list to master first. If your goal is to gain more flexibility, then your focus will be on flexibility and agility to begin with. If your flexibility is inhibiting your ability to do other types of exercise, then clearly you should prioritise flexibility or include it in your routine. Once you have decided on the skills that need improving, you can go back to your preferences from the questions above and decide on the type of workout that is going to work for you. If endurance is an important skill for you to master, but you are a bit fair weather with your exercise (like me) and running during the winter is out of the question, you are better off on a treadmill at a gym, an indoor exercise bike or rowing machine, or attending a dance class (with a friend if you need the accountability).

2. FITNESS WISDOM

An interesting thing that I've noticed about failing in achieving fitness, more so than any other area, is that people do not seem to learn from their mistakes. In other areas, such as business, academic study, or relationships, people look for patterns so that they don't make the same mistakes again. For example, below is a common conversation with a client.

Client: *"Every week, I think 'I need to sort it out'. I start my exercise routine, but as soon as anything goes wrong or I feel upset about something, I stop. I procrastinate and feel such great urges to eat. And only crisps, or chocolate will do!"*

Me: *"Think about what you were feeling at the time you decided not to workout and instead grabbed the chocolate. What is causing this pattern of behaviour?"*

Client: *"I need to be stricter about protecting my time. There is always something that gets in the way of my routine, like a birthday, or when we go on holiday. Then it's harder to go back to exercising and being sensible. Once I stop exercising and eat the wrong thing, it's a free for all."*

But what is the context? This client sees skipping a few work-outs and eating without self-control as totally messing up.

They see themselves as a failure without any underlying context.

By practising more self-awareness, this client eventually broke down her behaviour of skipping workouts and binging into discrete events and related them back to the decisions that were made. We objectively agreed that skipping a week of workouts is hardly a slip up. The next time this client sees this same pattern, she can use previous experiences to disrupt her usual course of action to try and prevent the same pattern. But life happens! The important part here is not quitting. It doesn't mean you have to "start again". You are simply carrying on where you left off.

Think of this self-awareness as *fitness wisdom*. It's the ability to learn more about yourself and your feelings. Without it, you wouldn't be able to learn from your mistakes.

3. PRACTICING SELF-COMPASSION

"What's wrong with me?"

Do you ever utter these words to yourself? I most certainly do and I have no idea where it came from! I stub my toe on the table and ask myself, *"What's wrong with me? How did I not see that table?"* But it can happen with the more serious stuff too, such as when it comes to achieving your goals, being resistant to stepping outside your comfort zone, and prioritising YOU.

So, why do we say these things to ourselves? First, we are assuming there is something wrong. Secondly, we assume this thing must be us. We are under so much pressure to be a "complete" woman -

- To balance everything
- Be interesting
- Be intelligent
- Have the perfect body
- Have the perfect home
- Be the perfect wife
- Be the perfect mother
- Be the perfect employee/business owner.

Is it surprising then, that you are left feeling like you are not enough? And this feeling rolls over into your efforts to get fit. You believe you are not doing enough, and what you are doing is not good enough. When you mess up on your diet, or fail to complete a single workout in weeks, the typical feelings you experience are hate, guilt, and self-loathing. You then feel the need to prove yourself, which leads you to doing all the work and feeling overwhelmed, underappreciated, and under-valued. You are also associating exercise with these negative feelings, so it's not surprising you don't want to do it. I see so many women feeling "less than", questioning their abilities (despite being very "successful"), and letting fear get in the way of stepping outside their comfort zones.

I see it so clearly because as a busy lawyer in a previous chapter of my life, a current business owner and mum, I have been through the exact same experiences and feelings. I have seen countless women who have never been able to lose, or maintain, a certain weight, and this perceived failure has created a lifetime of negative feelings. Yet they keep trying, over and over again, often relying on willpower to overcome their deficiencies. Each time, they face the same disastrous outcome.

We know that the solution is to think of fitness as a skill (not a talent) that has to be practiced in the right way, and research has shown that developing self-compassion allows you to do just that.[3] Those who show self-compassion forgive themselves for their mistakes so that they can try again - like you did as a child when you were learning to ride your bike. As a skill, it is not something we innately know how to do. Getting help from experts can help us improve the skills required in the most effective way. When it comes to fitness, the skill of self-compassion allows you to stop and think before you dive headfirst into the Ben & Jerry's ice-cream and ask yourself, "*Is this going to help fuel my body for better health?*" Or, when it comes to your exercise, "*Is my negative self-talk during this workout going to help me complete it?*" Self-compassion helps you to cut yourself some slack, then take the time to figure out what went wrong, or turn yourself into your biggest cheerleader.

The kindest thing to do is to learn to love your body and accept that you can only control the controllables. This makes you stronger. You CAN achieve anything you set your mind to. You are enough. There is nothing wrong with you.

YOUR TENDENCY & YOUR FITNESS SKILLS

Let's look at how best you can develop your fitness skills alongside your Tendency.

TENDENCY	SKILL	TAKEAWAY
Upholder	• You are disciplined when it comes to creating new habits, so use this ability to develop the physical skills needed for exercise. • Follow a structured plan - you can achieve great success with only a little guidance. • Practice showing some self-compassion and ditch the perfectionism.	Harness your natural discipline to develop physical skills and some self compassion.
Questioner	• With your goal in mind, decide which skills you need to master to help you choose the right workout plan. • But don't overthink your workout plan. Choose something that you feel is right for you and stick with it. • Accept that you may need to work on skills that you do not perceive to be central to your goals, in order to achieve success.	Consistency is key. Don't over analyse the process - stick with it.
Obliger	• Your best resource is to find a structure of accountability. Be clear on the type of accountability that is going to work for you. • Establish clear boundaries with those around you. This is a skill that is important for your success.	Your top skill is seeking the right accountability to sustain your exercise habit. You need the support.
Rebel	• Choose a physical skill that most appeals to you. You thrive on novelty, unconventionality and extremes, so choosing a form of exercise that sets you apart from others can work well. • Don't let others pressure you - be your unique self in the world of fitness.	Be your unique and creative self and choose the exercise regime that makes you feel good.

CHAPTER SUMMARY

- Our bodies are all different and we will have different aptitudes and capabilities in terms of movements that we can do, or do easily.

- But movement and exercise - and hence, fitness - are skills that we can practice and improve - yet we often seem to forget that.
- We need to work on the various components of these skills to get better at them - your physical skills (types of exercise, how much and when); fitness or wisdom mindset (attitude and self-belief); self-compassion (forgiving your mistakes, learning from them and trying again); and discipline (sticking with it through initial hardship to develop fitness habits that become easy to maintain).
- Start by focusing on what may be affecting your ability to follow through on these 5 components - is it time, money, physical capability, mental effort, or impact on your routine that is causing the blockage?
- Once you know the key problem(s), you can focus on resolving it/them, so that your circumstances are optimised to allow you to succeed.

NEXT STEPS

EVIDENCE JOURNAL

This is a little like the Greatest Hits list you created in Chapter 3, but this time you are going to track and make a list of the actual exercise you achieved each day / week. I find it's easier to track each day by spending 5 minutes in the evening noting them down. You can use a table similar to the one below, or make a record in your journal. Think about:

1. The particular form of movement you achieved. This doesn't need to be a formal workout. This can be any type of movement that you have done during your day that has benefitted your body. For example, choosing to take the stairs rather than the escalator, doing 10 press ups before your lunch, balancing on a wobble board while you wait for the kettle to boil, dancing around your kitchen, going for a walk etc.
2. Next, make a note of how each movement / workout made you feel.

This evidence journal will help you to gather evidence of you using your skills and capabilities when it comes to movement and positively reinforcing the experience by focusing on how good it made you feel. Not only will this lead you to become more aware of your movement patterns each day (it can be quite shocking how long we spend sitting each day), but it will also help you be more creative in finding new ways to move in alignment with your goals. Remember, if your goal is to strengthen your body, you need to incorporate the skills of strength, stamina and agility into your workouts from the list at the beginning of this chapter.

WHEN	WHAT EXERCISE	HOW LONG	HOW YOU FELT

14

WHERE TO GO FROM HERE

A s you will have realised from this book, there is no single universal solution that exists to get you to exercise on a regular basis. It is a unique experience for each and every one of us. Only when you start to become more self-aware can you begin to make necessary changes in your life, and this is particularly true for fitness. I have included an example Map to Success in the **Appendix**, so you can see how to structure your own, based on the exercises you have completed in this book. It's a useful resource to refer back to when life gets challenging. It's the map that can give you a kick up the butt when you need it, or an opportunity to demonstrate self-compassion through the words you have written. If you have read through this book without completing the Next Steps tasks after each chapter, I urge you to go back and complete them. It is the work *you* do that will make the real difference.

At the start, your goal isn't to judge yourself or feel guilty about your behaviours up to this point. You are exactly where you're meant to be right now. Having read this book and participated in the thought exercises and other tasks, you are now armed with a better understanding of who you are and what works for you, as well as a variety of strategies to move you towards your fitness goals.

Be curious. Try them out, and if they don't work, try some more. Take your time to really explore who you are and what makes you tick. Eventually you will discover which strategies work for you. It may require some imagination and it will most certainly require you to step out of your comfort zone occasionally. But when this happens, you know you are making progress. No more dreaming about how you would like things to be when you eventually have some time on your hands (which we know is never going to happen). It is awareness that will show you how to make the change you know you need to embrace. Armed with more knowledge about your Tendency and the strategies that are best suited to you can help set you up to keep making small daily changes.

We are all a work in progress. Learning to exercise regularly is a cyclical path, not a linear one. There is no beginning and end, but rather a constant flow of learning, changing, sometimes failing, sometimes succeeding. You are human and have emotional responses to what life throws at you and this will, on occasion, necessitate a different approach to your self-care practices. Life will happen and you will experience ups and downs - and some of those downs will completely knock you off course. Your job is to roll with those times. Like the weather, you can't change it. But we can learn to wait for the rain to pass and the clouds to clear, as we know they will. You have the power to make the necessary change and create a habit of exercise. I truly believe that as we grow older, our bodies should continue to improve, not stagnate, or deteriorate. It is within your power, knowledge, and experience to future-proof the wonderful body you have, in order to live a long, happy, and healthy life.

And of course I can't finish this book without espousing the health benefits of dance. From the age of two I have danced and intend to continue for as long as my body will allow me to do so. Yes, dance provides a multitude of physical benefits, but it is how it makes you feel that means once you start it is forever a part of you. It changes the way you move and your relationship with your physical surroundings. It also activates your cognitive pathways to change the way you think, solve problems and take risks, as well as enhancing spatial awareness and mental agility.[1] As Dr Peter Lovatt says;

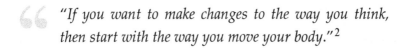
"If you want to make changes to the way you think, then start with the way you move your body."[2]

My sincere wish is that by using this book, you will gain a deeper understanding of your mind and body to help you set and implement exercise goals and begin to truly understand the benefits of movement to your overall physical, mental, and emotional wellbeing. Let this book be the catalyst for a lifelong habit of daily movement in whatever form that takes. Be proud of how far you have already come since starting this book. Remember, you are looking at making a 1% improvement each day. It is doable and you are more than capable. Just imagine how your life is going to feel in six months' time, or in two years, or ten years. I'm excited for you! For now, it's time to MOVE!

FOR MORE INFORMATION ABOUT BREAKING BALLET:

21 Day Body Re-Boot

To help kickstart your exercise regime from the comfort of your own home, visit https://breakingballet.com/body-re-boot/ for 21 days of ballet-inspired workouts, and meal plans. This body and mind workout programme is specifically designed for women in their 40s and beyond. That means it's designed specifically for YOUR body and YOUR hormones.

Best Body Journal

A useful journal to help record your health and fitness progress. Visit https://breakingballet.com/journal/ to purchase your copy.

Connect with Sarah and find out more about Breaking Ballet:

hello@breakingballet.com www.breakingballet.com www.facebook.com/breakingballet www.instagram.com/breakingballet/ www.youtube.com/c/BreakingBallet

APPENDIX

YOUR MAP TO SUCCESS

Throughout this book you have been mapping out your key personal strategies that will help you create a sustainable habit of exercise. The following is a worked example of what your map to success might look like.

You will need to revisit this map from time to time to update your strategies, such as your process goals. For example, once you have created a habit of drinking more water each day, you may want to start focusing on eating a healthy breakfast each morning to further support your progress towards your destination goal. You may also want to change your focus slightly in relation to old habits when you have successfully removed some of them. Also, once you have achieved your destination goal, your map will need to be updated with your new goal, along with your new process goals.

EXAMPLE MAP TO SUCCESS
KATY: OBLIGER

THE KEY PARTS	MY STRATEGIES	*WHY THEY WORK*
TENDENCY	I'm an Obliger. My key characteristics are: 1. I meet outer expectations easily. 2. I feel a sense of obligation to others. 3. I'm susceptible to burnout because of my people pleasing nature.	*Knowing your Tendency gives you greater self-awareness and helps you to shape your goals and strategies for success in ways that work for your unique personality.*
STRENGTHS AND WEAKNESSES	My Strengths 1. I'm organised. 2. I am friendly and loyal. 3. I am determined to succeed (provided I have support in doing so). My Weaknesses 1. I'm easily distracted away from my goals by other people. 2. I lack confidence and can sometimes give up if I don't feel what I'm doing is good enough. 3. I'm impatient and can sometimes expect results to come sooner than is perhaps realistic.	*You can take these from the "Gaining Self-Awareness" exercise on Strengths and Weaknesses in Chapter 2.*

THE KEY PARTS	MY STRATEGIES	*WHY THEY WORK*
KEY MOTIVATORS = 1. **MY WHY** 2. **MY GREATEST HITS**	1. To be a good role model for my children. 2. My work presentation last month. Training for and running a 10k race 10 years ago. Revising for and passing school exams. Coaching others at work. Meeting work deadlines.	*1. Katy has a need to be a good role model and finds it difficult to exercise for her benefit only.* *2. These Greatest Hits will change her thought processes but will also be a useful evidence log of all the times she has been successful in motivating herself to complete a task.* *Katy completed the journaling task in Chapter 3 to help her reflect on her life and the times she succeeded in achieving particular goals, so she is able to better understand what can motivate her to exercise.*
MY KEY BELIEFS ("I CAN BECAUSE…")	I can exercise because I deserve to practice self-care - I'm worth it. I can exercise regularly because I'm strong and capable.	*Katy is reframing her limiting beliefs (not feeling worthy of self-care and not having the physical strength to achieve her goals,) so she can better choose how to behave to create new habits that will support and reinforce her exercise identity.*
MY KEY VALUES (TOP 8)	• Health • Family / Friends • Balance • Energy • Confidence • Longevity • Fun • Positivity	*Katy's goals are now in alignment with her core values.* *She places high value on meeting commitments to others, so now she knows she needs to find outer accountability to achieve her goals.*

THE KEY PARTS	MY STRATEGIES	*WHY THEY WORK*
MY DESTINATION GOAL	I want to complete a 5k run. This will help me to lose weight (I'm aiming for 1 stone) and improve my cardiovascular fitness and stamina (at the moment I'm out of breath when I get to the top of the stairs). This improved fitness and weight loss will make me feel happier, stronger and more energised. I will be showing my children that it's important to prioritise your health and wellbeing.	*Now Katy has a base on which to build her process goals to help her achieve this one big goal.* *She knows what her "why" is - she used the "Painting a picture" exercise in Chapter 3 to help her gain clarity around this.* *She has also applied the SMART goals to ensure this goal will work for her.*
MY PROCESS GOALS TO CREATE MY HABIT OF EXERCISE (3 NON-NEGOTIABLES)	1. Complete a 15 minute workout each morning - a combination of running (3 x per week), strength training (2 x per week) and stretching (2 x per week) (Move) - I will lay out my workout clothes the night before and ensure I have decided which workout I'm doing the next day and have my exercise space ready/trainers at the door. 2. Drink 8 glasses of water a day (Nourish). I'm going to track my water intake in my journal, fill a water bottle on my desk and also set an alarm on my phone to remind	*Katy has applied the same SMART principles to set her process goals and also looked at her "why" to help her take action on these goals every day.* *This is just the start and if Katy feels these process goals are too much to begin with she can reduce the timescales, or switch them out into something more manageable.* *Once she is running for 15 minutes, she can increase her runtime to 20 minutes - building it up incrementally by 5 minutes at a time over the weeks.* *Achieving these simple goals each day is sustainable and will make Katy feel like she's*

THE KEY PARTS	MY STRATEGIES	WHY THEY WORK
	me to drink because I never really feel thirsty so I need the reminder. 3. Go to bed at 10pm every night (Nurture). Turn off my phone before going to the bedroom, or leave it in the kitchen. I will set an alarm to remind me to start my evening routine earlier. I have a new book which is making going to bed seem more attractive as this is time for me.	*finally prioritising herself. This will give her a sense of calm and wellbeing so she is no longer feeling stressed and overwhelmed with life. Exercise will start to feel like a treat, rather than a chore.* *She will ask a friend to keep her accountable with her goals because she knows this accountability is important for her success.* *She has put steps in place to make her new habits obvious, attractive, easy and satisfying.*
OLD HABITS I'M DITCHING	1. Hitting the snooze button in the morning when my alarm goes off. I will move my alarm clock to the other side of the room so I have to get up to turn it off. Once I'm up, I'm up! 2. Snacking on treats mid-afternoon. I will remove all treats from the house because I have realised I'm much more likely to succeed if I remove temptation altogether. I will place a bowl of fruit in the middle of the kitchen that I have to walk past. I will tell myself that if I'm not hungry enough to eat a piece of fruit, I don't	*Making the habits invisible, unattractive, difficult and unsatisfying will help Katy to stop doing them. She will have strategies in place to ensure she keeps working towards her goals.*

THE KEY PARTS	MY STRATEGIES	WHY THEY WORK
	need to eat anything. 3. Eating dinner too late at night. I will eat with the children at 6pm (or by 7pm latest if I'm working), rather than leaving it until 9pm.	
WHAT'S THE COST OF CONTINUING THESE OLD HABITS?	If I continue to snack and not workout I'm going to gain weight. The sweet treats also affect my blood sugar balance, leading to energy slumps and more snacking to counteract this feeling.	*Katy recognises that if she continues with these habits she's never going to achieve her goal of feeling strong and fit and full of energy. In fact, she will be achieving the exact opposite.*
WHAT WILL TRIP ME UP?	Having snacks and sweet treats available to me when I'm not at home. Being on holiday and out of routine, which may mean I don't get up in time to do my early morning workout. Not having the accountability I need. My friend might get bored of checking in on me.	*Katy knows I she will need to use the power of distraction if this circumstance arises. She can also revisit her "why" before giving into the craving.* *She can choose to let go of her exercise regime while on holiday for a week or so. It's ok to do this and doesn't mean she has "fallen off the wagon". She will continue with her routine as soon as she's home.* *If the accountability doesn't work with her friend, her plan B is to ask her partner to help, or join a community of women (on or offline) to help support her in reaching her goals.*

THE KEY PARTS	MY STRATEGIES	*WHY THEY WORK*
MY IDENTITY - WHO DO I NEED TO BE TO ACHIEVE MY GOAL?	I am an exerciser - I exercise daily. I prioritise my health and fitness and take good care of my body.	*Katy has told people about her decision to alter this aspect of her identity which will help her stick to her habits.* *If she needs to, she will join a group of like-minded women to maintain her habits.* *She knows that friendship and community will help her to embed this new identity.*
HOW MY PHYSICAL ENVIRONMENT WILL SUPPORT ME	I will sign a written commitment statement and share this with my friend. I will have a copy of this stuck to my fridge door to remind me of how to stay accountable. I will track my progress goals in a journal to support the accountability I receive from my friend. I will set up my workout space in the corner of the living room - creating an exercise "zone" just for me.	*Katy understands that making her commitment to exercise visible to those around her is an important factor supporting her to achieve her goals. So she will also share her goals with her family and friends.*
HOW MY SOCIAL ENVIRONMENT WILL SUPPORT ME	Using my friend for support and accountability feels good. When my confidence grows I will join a group of like-minded women so I can share this fitness journey with a wider group. I'm going to view my body as my best friend and treat it differently as a result. When I feel like skipping a	*Katy is mindful of choosing the right accountability for her. At the moment she doesn't want to get a personal trainer, or attend a gym. Her friend's support is enough and she plans on branching out a little when her confidence grows.*

THE KEY PARTS	MY STRATEGIES	*WHY THEY WORK*
	workout I will know that I'm letting my body down (as well as my commitment to my friend).	
BOUNDARIES I WILL PUT IN PLACE TO PROTECT MY EXERCISE HABIT	Saying "no" more often will stop me from overcommitting to others, leaving me with little time to prioritise my own needs. Telling my friends and family about my new identity and my goals will help to manage their expectations when it comes to the demands placed on my time.	*Katy's not good at saying "no" but ends up feeling resentful and exhausted and not having any time to prioritise her health and wellbeing. This has to stop. She knows that no-one else can do this for her. She's responsible for taking care of herself and she will ensure she has the outer accountability she needs to achieve her goals.*
WHAT EVIDENCE DO I HAVE THAT I'M EXERCISING?	I am going to keep an exercise journal and spend 5 minutes each evening writing down all the exercise I have done that day (including non exercise physical activity).	*Tracking her progress will help to keep her focused. She can share this record with her friend to show her compliance with her commitment statement.*

REFERENCES

1. THINK BEFORE YOU MOVE

1. British Heart Foundation; Women and heart diseasehttps://www.bhf. org.uk/informationsupport/heart-matters-magazine/medical/ women/coronary-heart-disease-kills
2. Royal Osteoporosis Society; What's the menopause got to do with bone health? https://theros.org.uk/blog/2021-03-22-what-s-the-menopause-got-to-do-with-bone-health/#:~:text=If%20you%20have%20an%20early,weaker%20bones%20in%20later%20life.
3. Williams, Caroline. Move - The New Science of Body Over Mind, (2021) Profile Books.
4. Lovatt, Peter. Dr. The Dance Cure - The surprising secret to being smarter, stronger, happier (2020) Short Books, p.99-103.

3. MOTIVATION TO MOVE

1. Pontzer, H. Burn - The Misunderstood Science of Metabolism (2021) Allen Lane, p258.
2. Fogg, BJ. Tiny Habits - The Small Changes that Change Everything (2019), Virgin Books, p137,
3. Pontzer, Herman. Burn - The Misunderstood Science of Metabolism (2021) Allen Lane, p259
4. Lieberman, D. Exercised - The Science of Physical Activity, Rest and Health, (2020) Penguin Random House, p256.

4. BELIEFS SHAPE YOUR REALITY

1. Inspired by James Murphy, Executive Coach, Founder of Evolution for Success, (2012) https://www.executivecoachinglifecoaching.com/nlp-behavior-patterns/

7. SMALL CHANGES MAKE THE BIGGEST DIFFERENCES

1. Dispenza, Dr Joe. Breaking the Habit of Being Yourself, (2012) Hay House UK Ltd
2. 1.01^{365} = 37.78 James Clear https://jamesclear.com/continuous-improvement
3. Rubin, Gretchen. Better Than Before - What I learned about making and breaking habits to sleep more, quit sugar, procrastinate less and generally build a happier life (2015), Two Roads, p201ff
4. Walker, M. Why We Sleep - The New Science of Sleep and Dreams (2017) Allen Lane, p.172.
5. Walker, M. Why We Sleep - The New Science of Sleep and Dreams (2017) Allen Lane, p.175.
6. https://melrobbins.com/5secondrule/
7. Walker, M. Why We Sleep - The New Science of Sleep and Dreams (2017) Allen Lane, p.43
8. Mel Robbins: Why hitting "snooze" ruins your brain https://www.youtube.com/watch?v=iwollxDAm0Y

9. EXERCISE IDENTITY

1. Is physical activity a part of who I am? A review and meta-analysis of identity, schema and physical activity Ryan E. Rhodes, Navin Kaushal &Alison Quinlan

    Pages 204-225 | Received 17 Aug 2015, Accepted 14 Jan 2016, Accepted author version posted online: 25 Jan 2016, Published online: 02 Mar 2016
2. https://www.researchgate.net/figure/Exercise-identity-The-main-branches-show-the-three-main-influences-on-exercise-identity_fig1_51472176
3. Strachan, S. & Stadig, G. (2015). I'm an exerciser. Common conceptualisations of and variation in exercise identity meanings. *International Journal and Exercise Psychology, 15*(3), 321-336.
4. Strachan, S. & Stadig, G. (2015). I'm an exerciser. Common conceptualisations of and variation in exercise identity meanings. *International Journal and Exercise Psychology, 15*(3), 321-336.

5. Rhodes, R. E., Kaushal, N., & Quinlan, A. (2016). Is physical activity a part of who I am? A review and meta-analysis of identity, schema, and physical activity. *Health Psychology Review, 10*(2), 204-225.
6. Clear, J. Atomic Habits - Tiny Changes, Remarkable Results (2018) Random House Business Books, p30.
7. Munroe-Chandler KJ, Guerrero MD. Psychological imagery in sport and performance. In: *Oxford Research Encyclopedia of Psychology.* Oxford University Press; 2017. doi:10.1093/acrefore/9780190236557.013.228
8. https://www.verywellfit.com/visualization-techniques-for-athletes-3119438#citation-4
9. Melanie G M, Perros, Shaelyn M. Strachan, Michelle S. Fortier, Possible Selves and Physical Activity in Retirees: The Mediating Role of Identity 2016 Nov;38(8):819-41. doi: 10.1177/0164027515606191. Epub 2015 Sep 24.

10. BECOME THE ARCHITECT OF YOUR BEHAVIOUR

1. Alexander, C. The Timeless Way of Building (1979) New York Oxford University Press, p106

11. SURROUND YOURSELF WITH THE RIGHT PEOPLE

1. Christakis, N A. and Fowler, J. H. The Spread of Obesity in a Large Social Network over 32 Years (2007) N Engl J Med 2007; 357:370-379
2. Rubin, Gretchin. Better Than Before - What I Learned About Making and Breaking Habits — to Sleep More, Quit Sugar, Procrastinate Less, and Generally Build a Happier Life (2015), p250

12. BODY AWARENESS

1. McManus S, Bebbington P, Jenkins R, Brugha T. (eds.) (2016) Mental health and wellbeing in England: Adult Psychiatric Morbidity Survey 2014. Leeds: NHS Digital. Available at: http://content.digital.nhs.uk/catalogue/PUB21748/apms-2014-full-rpt.pdf

2. Weaver, L. Dr. Rushing Woman's Syndrome (2017) Hay House UK Ltd
3. https://www.theguardian.com/lifeandstyle/2022/jun/29/move-your-self-happy-how-to-exercise-boost-mood-fitness-level?
4. Williams, Caroline. Move - The New Science of Body Over Mind (2021), Profile Books.

13. DISCOVERING HOW CAPABLE YOU REALLY ARE

1. Fogg, BJ. Tiny Habits - The Small Changes That Change Everything (2019) Virgin Books
2. Rubin, Gretchin. Better Than Before - What I Learned About Making and Breaking Habits — to Sleep More, Quit Sugar, Procrastinate Less, and Generally Build a Happier Life (2015) Two Roads, p62
3. https://www.heidigranthalvorson.com/2012/09/forget-self-esteem.html

14. WHERE TO GO FROM HERE

1. Lovatt, Peter. Dr. The Dance Cure - The surprising secret to being smarter, stronger, happier (2020) Short Books, p76.
2. Lovatt, Peter. Dr. The Dance Cure - The surprising secret to being smarter, stronger, happier (2020) Short Books, p120.

Lightning Source UK Ltd.
Milton Keynes UK
UKHW022135241022
411033UK00010B/541/J